Beautiful LIGHT

Overcoming Severe Anorexia

Memoir & Collective

CASSANDRA ALANE

IMPRESSUM

PRAISE for *Beautiful Light*

"*Beautiful Light* is a powerful journey of resilience and recovery. Authored by a survivor, it offers invaluable insights, practical strategies and compassionate guidance for those battling anorexia. With a blend of personal anecdotes and lived expertise, this book is a beacon of hope, highlighting the path towards self-love and healing. Its empathetic approach fosters understanding and empowers individuals to embrace nourishment, both physically and emotionally. *Beautiful Light* is not just a book; it's a lifeline for anyone navigating the turbulent waters of anorexia, offering solace and strength on the road to recovery."

Alison Buttenshaw,
Author of *Out of the Shadows*, Lived Experience and Life Coach

"As a nurse who has cared for people with eating disorders and educated clinicians in treating people with eating disorders for many years, *Beautiful Light* has reminded me that above all, 'holding the hope' is the most important message we must give our patients, their families and the health professionals who will at times when dealing with anorexia feel utterly hopeless. Cassandra is honest, optimistic and generous, as she shares her experiences and insights focusing on the whole person, and this is where her spirituality is felt by the reader. It is my privilege to have read Cassandra's book, and I wholeheartedly recommend *Beautiful Light.*"

Bridget Mulvey,
Clinical Nurse Consultant for Eating Disorders at InsideOut Institute, Sydney

"Cassandra's story is a brave, honest, heartfelt and ultimately hopeful message for all who suffer with an eating disorder and those who provide care and support. Her spirituality is a beacon of light that literally emanates throughout and in doing so, reinforces for the reader the possibility of social and emotional wellbeing. A personal and profoundly resonating book I am proud to endorse and recommend."

Bronny Caroll,
Carer and Advocate for Eating Disorders

"An amazing resource for anyone wanting to understand more about anorexia. I highly recommend *Beautiful Light* to individuals tormented by an eating disorder and to those desperately trying to help. I too have recovered, in my case, from bulimia. Like Cassandra, I know the importance of feeling heard, understood and not alone and that hope, healing and life can be found. Cassandra is brave to share her story and struggles while offering true hope, practical steps and an anchor to hold on to. I believe this book will bless anyone who reads it."

Maxine Vorster,
Author of *Hidden Hunger*, Inspirational Speaker and Christian Counsellor,
Switzerland

"I loved reading, *Beautiful Light*. It was so raw and real, but mostly for me, as a general practitioner, it helped me to understand a patient's perspective much better than I ever had before. Thank you, Cassandra, for being so honest and raw; and for the hope you offer all sufferers that this illness can be overcome. May your future always remain bright."

Doctor Libby Sutton,
General Practitioner, Atune Health Centre, Newcastle

Beautiful Light

To my family, friends and the health professionals who journeyed with
me, your care made a world of difference—thank you. And to all those
with anorexia and the people who support them,
I dedicate *Beautiful Light* to you.

CONTENTS

FOREWORD

Cassandra is an incredible person. I knew that as soon as I met her. I have since learnt that every person I have met who has managed to recover from anorexia nervosa once it has persisted for a time, is an incredible person. Recovering from anorexia nervosa is nothing short of a sheer act of personal will, determination, creativity and life force. I know in Cassandra's case, she feels she was helped enormously by spiritual forces; everyone who has to go through this, I hope, is assisted by every force that can come to their aid.

Cassandra has taught me many things. Perhaps the most important to my own life is that no matter the circumstances, no matter the predictions, no matter the dire medical and psychological situation, one can, if the right circumstances prevail, recover from this deadly illness.

She was the first patient I treated as a young intern and then registered psychologist, and for better or worse, she set me on the path that would become my career, and from her experience and strength imparted to me an unwavering (so far!) belief in hopefulness.

Cassandra worked extremely hard over many years, and I did too. I was only one of the people in her care team and her life who willed her along, tried hard to devise new strategies and treatment options, persisted and hung in there just as she hung in there and waited for the change in circumstances or opportunities and forged forward again.

It has been one of the greatest joys life affords to see her recover, grow, flourish and build her life, friendships, family, work and passions. She is in every way an inspiration, and I hope this book allows many more people to understand that and to share in the hope and light Cassandra brings.

Prof Sarah Maguire, OAM
Clinical Psychologist and Director of InsideOut Institute, Sydney

INTRODUCTION

I was just seventeen years old when they transferred me to an adult psychiatric unit with severe anorexia. It was the fourth treatment facility I had been in. I was an involuntary patient, and recovery was not something I wanted or could even allow myself to think about. Eating disorder rules, fear and the effects of starvation consumed and controlled my every thought, feeling and action. Simple pleasures—laughter, rest and human touch—were things of the past. I was unreachable, detached from people, the world around me and even my own heart. Any glimmer of hope in finding freedom and a life worth living was far gone.

A single spiritual encounter, however, turned all of this around. Instantly, I went from having no hope to finding hope. Hope because my soul found what it longed for. Hope because I felt seen, safe and understood. With rays of light now shining through, freedom began to appear, and with good support, the path to complete and sustainable recovery opened before me.

As a result, I have a message to share: "Yes, it is difficult for someone with anorexia to find what enables them to move and keep moving towards recovery. Difficult, but not impossible."

Beautiful Light, therefore, seeks to impart hope where there may seem to be none. Hope that light can break through, inner life can be found and the road to recovery can prove absolutely worthwhile. At the same time, through sharing my story and discoveries, *Beautiful Light* also offers insight into anorexia, spirituality and recovery—uplifting a holistic way forward.

So, let's take a little walk through *Beautiful Light*.

Upon entering my story at *Daybreak*, you will find recovery is not just about food and weight. We then step back into my childhood. Thankfully, I did not have anorexia as a child. Nonetheless, exploring these foundational years helps us to understand aspects of the disorder and importantly—the person underneath it all.

From here, we move to *Sunset*, where as a preteen, poor self-image and feelings of sadness, anger and shame set in. Everything then changes when I look to dieting for help. Anorexia rapidly takes hold, and professional help steps in at *Dusk*. All the while, my innermost needs remain unmet. Pressing forward through A *Long Night*, I share my thoughts, fears and struggles (being mindful to provide insight without elevating the detrimental aspects of anorexia). You will see how consuming, tormenting and controlling the disorder is and what enables me to find life-giving hope amidst it all.

Awakening comes next, where the spiritual path unfolds, lighting the way forward through the mental, emotional and near-physical death anorexia brings, which takes us to *Dawn*. Holistic recovery surfaces here with professional help, family, friends and spirituality. At *Sunrise*, complete recovery emerges. I navigate challenges and life continues to break through. *A New Day* then begins. However, this is not where I show you a picture-perfect life. Instead, it is where you see what life looks like beyond anorexia—and it isn't dull. Passion, purpose, failings, heartache and delight all colour my life. I am free to live in the moment, and on the other side of anorexia, I realise just how precious this is.

Venturing further, we come to *The Ray Collective*. Here, I gather poetry, stories, journal entries and letters into four easy-to-read chapters, along with the best insights and most inspiring messages I have on understanding and overcoming anorexia. For instance, I share how recovery does not necessarily equate to returning to our old selves and lives, as the term implies. Rather, we can discover new dimensions of our identity and a better reality beyond the disorder. You will also find I write from a Christian perspective but that my writing is accessible to people of all beliefs and highlights how integral spirituality can be in a person's journey.

In brief, *The Ray Collective's* first chapter, *Looking Within,* offers insight into how the disorder can develop and impact the body and soul. We then enter *Finding Hope,* which explores the spiritual path and how it can supply our soul needs. Following on, *Holistic Recovery* shows how professional help, family, friends and spirituality can support complete recovery. Lastly, *Beyond Anorexia* reveals what positive and sustainable change can look like, physically, mentally and emotionally—instilling hope and diminishing fear for the journey ahead.

For people with anorexia, I believe, along with finding a story of hope, you'll be able to identify with aspects of my journey and take away rays of light that speak to you. These rays may appear as edifying truths, encouragement to seek help, inspiration to keep going or simply comfort in knowing you are not alone. At the same time, *Beautiful Light* affirms the unique path each person is on. It recognises no two people—and therefore no two recovery stories—are alike. So, my experience isn't a one-size-fits-all antidote. Instead, I share my journey to encourage and empower you wherever you find yourself. You will also discover my story helps others to see that the person behind anorexia has not only a body but a soul and a spirit. I hope this serves you well.

For carers and health professionals, *Beautiful Light* will enhance and perhaps even challenge your understanding of anorexia and how spirituality can assist recovery. It will also offer insight into holistic care and practical guidance on providing support. Journeying with me through my dark times, recovery and beyond will also help stir empathy and fresh hope. And while you will see not all treatment or care offered was beneficial or accepted—unconditional love, understanding and patience from those offering support prevailed. So, I hope you leave feeling inspired that while it may not always appear so, the care and support you show is indeed valuable, appreciated and much needed.

Ultimately, I have written *Beautiful Light* to shine hope and cultivate understanding. No one is beyond help, and everyone is worthy of it. Irrespective of how bleak it may seem, there is an incredible path full of life before each of us. So, whether you have anorexia, provide support or simply seek to learn and be inspired, I invite you to read my story with this in mind:

The skies may be cloudy, and the nights long,
yet beautiful light continues to shine.

Important Note

While this book is pro-recovery, it details my experience of anorexia, which may be unsettling for some. If this applies to you, I invite you to skip ahead to the *Resource* section and read the rest when ready. For parents, as *Beautiful Light* is written for a wide audience, I suggest reading it before deciding whether it's appropriate for your teen. If you have anorexia, you may even want to read *Beautiful Light* with your therapist or support person so you can discuss any issues raised, as well as the central message of hope.

Cassandra's Story

A Journey Into and Out of Severe Anorexia

1. Daybreak

Agitated, I sat on the edge of my bed in the adult psychiatric unit. I was eighteen years old, and I'd just completed my first expressive art project—a collage of my childhood. Nurse Jaine was keen to talk with me about it. Sitting and connecting with my feelings felt almost unbearable. It wasn't something the eating disorder allowed me to do, but she was as gentle as she was persistent.

"Can you point to a photo and explain it to me?"

"This is my dog, Jessie," I said, avoiding her eyes.

She nodded. "Why did you choose this one?"

"I … I love animals."

She pointed to another photo. In it, three smiling girls held star-printed balloons.

"Who are these lovely people?"

"That's my best friend Tanya and her little sister at my seventh birthday party."

"And this photo of the lady and baby?"

"That's my mum," I said. "Holding me."

Detached from self for so long through anorexia, reflecting on my upbringing felt dreamlike. It was as though I was looking at someone else's memories—but I knew they were mine. As I meditated on each photo, my soul began to stir, and I identified with parts of my life long forgotten.

Early Years

Classic homemade silent movies show Mum and Dad playing barefoot in the yard with our dog, Fella, and me sitting as an infant, patting our cats, Tibby, Toby and Tabby. Mum was known for her beauty, bohemian style and kind nature, while Dad was a salesperson with a gift for playing guitar and fixing cars. Named Cassandra, or Cassie for short, I was their first and only child, born into a middle-class family on the outskirts of Sydney in the 1980s.

Dad had another daughter from an earlier relationship. We didn't see each other much growing up; our sister bond formed later in life. So, I cherished the one photo I had of us from childhood, taken by a horse paddock. We also didn't live near our extended family, and since Mum was adopted, we hadn't met all our relatives yet. Nevertheless, we all shared one strong family trait—a love of animals.

Although Mum and Dad looked happy on the surface, all was not well. They divorced when I was just two years old. From there, I only saw Dad every second weekend. During that time, I also became sick with fevers and urinary infections, often looking quite jaundiced and was diagnosed with renal reflux. On top of the renal disorder, I experienced painful ear infections despite having grommets inserted. If that weren't enough for Mum to manage, I also developed asthma.

Somehow, amongst the break-up of our family and my sickness, Mum found faith in God, and we began attending church. Dad, on the other hand, already believed in God. Although he didn't take me to church,

Dad taught me to say grace and bedtime prayers, adding to my spiritual foundation and our father-daughter connection.

From a young age, Tanya was another significant person in my life. One of my most vivid early childhood memories is of us two. Mum recollected to other parents at my third birthday party, "Remember how Cassie bit Tanya at her party last year? I felt terrible when—"

Loud tears erupted, cutting her sentence short.

Admittedly, I had bitten Tanya *for the second year running*. A grown-up had asked me to be a good little girl and put away a toy. Tanya, however, had picked it up and put it away first. She was praised for doing so. It didn't seem right to me, so with a toddler's sense of injustice and a rush of anger, I bit her. Consequently, I was reprimanded for my behaviour and left with a lasting imprint of my overwhelming emotions.

Mum later brought me to a field with horses. "Only horses bite," she said. "Not little girls."

Sadly, the following year, Mum's adoptive father, Pa, became terminally ill and passed away. I have fond memories of Pa. He grew big bunches of spinach in his veggie patch and sat at the head of the dining table to carve the Sunday roast, which Ma, Mum's adoptive mother, baked. I also enjoyed wrapping my arms around his leg as he raised it up and down like a ride.

Mum worked through losing Pa with the support of neighbours and church friends while caring for me with renal reflux. After several doctor appointments, they decided I needed corrective surgery. Leading up to the procedure, I had an invasive, traumatic and humiliating test. I didn't want the test but being a child—I had no choice. Post-op, I was restricted to my bed with drips and a drain, which only added to my embarrassment.

A few days later, the girl in the hospital bed beside me was celebrating her birthday. I joined the celebration, but I didn't eat any cake, play or even smile. I sat with my arms crossed and was apparently "grumpy." Yet what I felt was anger and shame.

Later that year, Mum arranged for me to have professional photos taken. She just wanted some special pictures of her four-year-old to hang on our walls. When I saw them, I thought, *I look like a boy, not a pretty girl.* I didn't have long hair, wasn't petite and didn't like any of my features. Unable to express my embarrassment, I told Mum, "I don't look nice. I don't want the photos hung up."

Mum disagreed and placed the photos on display.

In the meantime, Dad had remarried, and in 1986, he and his new wife welcomed a baby girl into the world. I now had a cute little sister, who I enjoyed singing lullabies to each visit. We soon became good play-mates and expert cubby house builders. I also found myself with a minia-ture shadow, following me wherever I went.

We flew kites and rode bikes as a family at Dad's too. And I loved the food his wife cooked. I also felt safe at his place when drifting to sleep at night. Whereas, at Mum's, I felt vulnerable and anxious lying in bed, knowing we didn't have a man around to protect us from intruders. Yet, going to Dad's also meant obeying different rules, fulfilling different ex-pectations and adapting to a different lifestyle. Moreover, it entailed doing a part of my life without the warmth and care of Mum around.

Living in a split family felt normal and good—but also hard. Conse-quently, my behaviour was split. I behaved perfectly at Dad's, but not at Mum's. I wanted to please both my parents all the time, but I couldn't.

On Mum's weekends, we continued attending church. I didn't like church. Being shy, I sat with Mum at morning tea instead of playing with other kids. I also refused to stand for the singing during the service. My re-fusal was partly because of shyness but also due to sensing the sacredness of worship. I thought, *If God is real, then singing to him is a big deal.* I wasn't going to stand and sing just because everyone else was.

I did like singing, however, just for fun. I enjoyed rehearsing an item with my Sunday school class to sing at a coming church event. Mum picked out a dress for me to wear for the occasion. I was used to Dad choosing what I would wear, but I always chose my own clothing at Mum's. Yet she insisted this time I wear my red dotted and frilly dress. I hated that dress. Stamping my foot, I protested, "I'm not wearing it!" I ended up wearing the dress but felt so self-conscious and angry at Mum that I refused to stand on stage to sing.

With the new year came the start of primary school. From day one, I loved kindergarten, especially show-and-tell. When my turn came for show-and-tell, I took in a green box where I had carefully placed my first letter from Africa. Mum and I had sent gifts to Ugandan children the previous Christmas and received this thank you note. I thought it was special.

It also turned out that Tanya (who I no longer thankfully bit!) and I were in the same class, and we soon befriended a pretty girl with golden-blonde hair, Dianna. Unknowingly, the three of us had just begun a lifelong friendship together.

Then, as a first grader, another relationship formed, a spiritual one. Standing on my front lawn, in the cool of the night, staring up into the sky, I reasoned, *God must be real. How else would all these stars exist?* Too shy and self-conscious to tell anyone I now believed in God and would like to be baptised, I quietly promised God, "I'll get baptised when I can swim without floaties." I was only seven years old and was sure he'd understand.

We attended a Baptist Church, so I couldn't partake in communion until I was baptised. Not only did I feel like the odd one out as they passed communion by me each service, but I also felt like I was letting

God down. I wondered, *Am I really a Christian?* Being young and timid, I didn't talk to anyone about my doubts but kept my questions to myself.

There were times, though, when I wasn't shy. In the winter of 1989, my friend Paula and I proudly and excitedly walked down the aisle as flower girls for my mum's and stepdad's wedding. I had known my stepdad since I was two years old and was truly fond of him.

Shortly after they married, I was hospitalised with meningitis. I spent my eighth birthday in the children's ward. A cleaner gave me a little toy panda. "I was in hospital as a child, and no one gave me a gift. I didn't want you to miss out," she softly explained. I never forgot her kindness. Mum and my stepdad also brought in gifts and a cake to celebrate. With great effort, I took a deep breath and blew out the candles (on my germ-proof, cling-wrapped cake). Being too sick to eat, I just watched the other kids enjoy my cake.

Once recovered, I returned to school. I still loved school—apart from sports. My coordination skills were almost non-existent. I felt bad and embarrassed, letting teams down when I missed the ball. Not surprisingly, I didn't play sports outside of school. Instead, I joined the Brownies. I didn't mind the Brownies, but felt shy and awkward trying to join in. What I enjoyed was having penfriends. After seeing an advertisement about starving children in Africa, I started sponsoring a girl in Ethiopia, Ayana. We wrote to each other often. Ayana impressed me by how she always started her letters with, "Praise be to God." Although she was only my age, she sounded so mature and optimistic, despite her challenging situation.

Near the end of the year, our family dog, Fella, who was old and unwell, had to be put down. I dearly missed Fella. To cheer me up, I was gifted a woolly black, over-the-top friendly puppy. I named my pup Jessie and loved her with all my heart.

Mum also signed me up for a summer camp. Standing before a totem pole at camp, with no one around, I whispered to God, "I believe in you." I hoped this would make me a Christian, even though I wasn't baptised. I felt disappointed—I didn't feel different, and I didn't instantly start reading my Bible or praying more.

I spent most of third grade either in hospital with asthma or at home having the nebuliser. Feeling sick became more familiar than feeling well, and I fell behind in school. Learning how to rule margins was particularly challenging. I didn't understand the point behind them, so I couldn't grasp how to draw them. I concluded margins were stupid. I always needed to know the "whys." It was also the first year that Tanya wasn't in my class. We still played together in the schoolyard and after school with Dianna, but I missed having Tanya in my class. I felt lost without her.

I still struggled to fit in with the kids at church too, until Amber came along. I was so happy that Amber befriended me. Now, I had a friend my age at church. We also played outside of church with our friend Paula. We had fun conducting blindfolded taste-testing games, spending countless hours playing Nintendo, climbing trees and cooling off in Paula's saltwater pool.

∞

Life was good for me, even amongst sickness—Mum, on the other hand, was having difficulties. She avoided crowded places, rested a lot and was slim. I didn't know it, but Mum had agoraphobia, chronic fatigue and anxiety. Somewhere in amongst this, she developed anorexia. Mum, however, kept her struggles to herself and put my needs first. At age nine, I felt loved and content, but those feelings were about to fade.

2. Sunset

"What did the teacher say?" I eagerly asked Mum as she returned home from the parent-teacher interview.

"Sweetie, they are stepping you down to the B grade class next year because you missed a lot of schooling."

Paving the Way

I was hospitalised with asthma during the holidays and discharged on the first day of the new school year. Determined to prove I could do well at school, I decided not to miss a day and study hard. I returned home, put on my uniform and went straight to school. I came first in my fourth grade class both mid and end-year. I learnt I could achieve anything that I set my mind to. I felt confident and daring. I wore dangly feather earrings to school, a yellow scarf in my hair and even had a boy "ask me out" (my reply was no, I secretly liked another boy). Most of all, I enjoyed being in the same class as Tanya once again.

Yet, despite everything going well at school, I started finding aspects of life difficult. I was becoming more self-aware, and for the first time, I felt embarrassed about my eating when an adult commented that I had almost completed a larger meal than my friend. Still hungry but suddenly ashamed of my eating, I left the last bit. I didn't know it then, but taking steroids for asthma further increased my appetite, and at school I started chewing on straws, pencils and even the cusps of my sleeves. I also felt nervous about how much I could eat at home for afternoon tea.

Amidst this, I was finding it hard that going to Dad's sometimes meant missing friends' birthday parties and sleepovers. It also bothered me how I saw him fortnightly, which felt overly structured rather than natural. At the same time, my mum and stepdad were having marriage difficulties, and I became angry that Mum was seeing a counsellor and couldn't just get over her problems. I didn't like myself when I was angry, but I couldn't control my anger. I now cried myself to sleep most nights and told Mum, from time to time, I felt "still." I didn't know what depression was or that it ran in my family, but it was low-grade depression I was describing. I also zoned out in anxiety-provoking situations and counted in a specific way the letters in words that people had spoken. Perhaps this was the start of obsessive-compulsive disorder (OCD).

Ditto for fifth grade. I topped the class and enjoyed school. Helping my stepdad with his balloon business was fun too. I loved decorating function rooms with him and receiving pocket money and McDonald's in return. It was also exciting that Mum found her biological mother. We learnt of our Aboriginal heritage and that our family are Wiradjuri people. We met some of Mum's Uncles and Aunties too, and heard stories of how they, including my Gran, were taken from their home and placed into foster care during the 1940s. Mum didn't find her biological father, but we did learn he was of Italian descent.

On the downside, my mum and stepdad separated. I felt both relieved and sad. Yet life was good, so when irritability popped up towards Mum, I thought I was a bad daughter and felt ashamed of myself. I also felt guilty, believing I was displeasing God. I didn't know that my mood was partly a sign of depression. Because of my eating habits and natural physical development, I also gained a little bit of weight. My weight was average for my height and age. I wasn't overweight but "solid."

At Christmas time, I travelled with Dad, his wife and my little sister to Alice Springs for a holiday. It was my first time on an aeroplane. I enjoyed looking out the window at the tiny houses below, and oddly enough, the aeroplane food impressed me. Spending time with relatives I rarely saw, like my big sister, was a highlight. Dining at my Uncle and Auntie's kiosk each morning was also a novelty. Sitting at breakfast, Dad announced his New Year's resolution, "I'm going on a diet." Looking at me, he light-heartedly asked, "Do you want to join me?"

I shook my head, "I'm okay, thanks." At this point, I felt fine about my weight.

Academically, I did well in sixth grade, and as always, I had fun and laughed with Tanya. Actually, I got too carried away playing around, and the teacher sent me out of the classroom a few times. I was having fun, but I was also discontent. I was discontent with primary school, ready to move on to high school, unhappy with areas of my homelife and un-settled within. As a preteen, I wanted something more from life. And with the further breakdown of my family and underlying depression, I no longer felt the security and contentment I did as a child.

Adding to this, I felt exposed and embarrassed when our class got weighed for a math activity, and I was one of the heavier girls. I now wore t-shirts over my swimmers. Clothes shopping became an unpleasant event. I was between child and adult sizes, so the clothes were tight and didn't fit my body shape. I had no idea clothing sizes varied from brand to brand. The fluorescent lights in the changing rooms didn't help, providing an unflattering reflection. I started to think, *I look fat and ugly*. Being annoyed with Mum at the shops, I further felt ugly inside. Ironically, shopping trips often ended with me eating a chocolate bar. One time, chocolate wasn't enough to make me feel better, so I cried and found something sharp to mark my skin with instead.

High school was a welcomed change. I liked the new challenges and having more independence. What I didn't like, however, was my appearance and continued lack of sporting ability. Both made me feel embarrassed and self-conscious. I had acne for the first time and was now at the higher end of the healthy spectrum weight-wise, and relatives unintentionally made discouraging and shaming comments. I didn't say anything. I just politely smiled while feeling like I wanted to curl up and hide. What I needed, though, was for them to protect my heart and to speak words of affirmation about who I am rather than comment on my appearance. When invited to parties and other social events, it now took me ages to get ready. On and off went outfits, followed by spending far too much time doing and re-doing my hair. Feeling unattractive and irritated, getting ready would often end with me announcing, "That's it, I'm not going anywhere!"

Then Tanya, who lived two doors up, moved away near the end of the year. That was a hard change. We kept in touch—but I missed her dearly. I now walked to the school bus stop alone. Along the way, self-critical and exaggerated thoughts began playing over in my mind. *My hair looks stupid, I look so fat, I have big pimples all over my face* and on and on they went.

Thankfully, before Tanya moved, we had formed joint friendships at school, so I had a new circle of friends to hang out with. My friends were creative, funny and easy to get along with. On weekends, we tie-dyed clothes, cooked meals to share, camped in my backyard, rode bicycles, ate pizza in the park and read *Dolly* magazines.

My favourite song this year was "Return to Innocence" by *Enigma*. It presented something intriguing and beautiful—a journey of finding peace and happiness, which resonated with my soul.

So, life was good on one level as a thirteen-year-old. Yet, on another level, I had discontentment, poor self-image and underlying sadness—signs that all was not well. In retrospect, it would have been helpful to receive wise counsel from a trusted adult or for someone to ask, "Are you okay?"

The following year, in 1995, Mum checked herself into a local psychiatric unit. I knew Mum was run down and needed time to rest and recoup. I felt genuinely surprised, however, to learn that she was in treatment for anorexia. I reasoned to myself, *Mum has always been slim. She never speaks of diets or weight, hardly exercises and seems to eat well. Perhaps I heard wrong?* My stepdad lived near my high school, so I stayed with him while Mum was in the psych unit. As I began adjusting to the fact that Mum was in treatment for anorexia, another challenge arose.

Jessie's health rapidly declined, and it was up to me to look after our sick dog. I cared for her until she died. We had a special bond. The night before she died, I was staying over at Tanya's house and dreamt that Jessie came up to me in bed and licked my face. I later discovered that when I dreamt of Jessie, my stepdad had found her curled up on my bed at his house. She wasn't allowed in my bedroom and had never done this before. Jessie dying the following day on returning to my stepdad's broke my heart.

My stepdad tried to cheer me up, "Can I get you pizza for dinner?"

"No thanks. I'm not hungry."

I took several days off from school and drew pictures of her until I felt okay.

A couple of months later, Mum discharged herself from treatment, and I returned home, assuming she was better.

After such a turbulent year, my stepdad treated me to a holiday in Cairns. We enjoyed our time away, snorkelling and exploring the Daintree rainforest, until my stepdad suddenly fell ill while white-water rafting. We flew home, and he went straight to the hospital. The doctor informed us he suffered a major heart attack and might not make it. My stepdad, however, wasn't giving up on life, and to our relief, he pulled through.

Once the summer break was over, I began the ninth grade. An advocate from World Vision visited our high school and talked about poverty overseas and how to help. My heart stirred, and I thought *I would like to work for an organisation like this in the future.* I believed life had meaning and purpose, but at age fourteen, going on fifteen, I was stuck in school and spent weekends alternating between my parents. Being free to explore and engage in something that caught my heart's desire seemed out of reach. So naturally, sitting in class one day, I ripped out a page of math work.

Unimpressed, my teacher asked, "What is going on?"

"This is a waste of time. People are dying in poor countries, and we're sitting here doing pointless algebra," I boldly replied, and was swiftly sent out of the classroom.

Around the same time, with a growing desire for something more out of life, I questioned a pastor of another church, "Am I really a Christian even though I'm not baptised? And can I join in communion?"

His answer to both was, "Yes." He explained, "Above all, God is interested in our hearts' response to him."

Although reassuring, it seemed like a nice concept rather than something real and life-changing.

So, life carried on as usual, until one afternoon when we heard a knock at the door. My stepdad was standing on the front porch with news to share, "I'm going to travel up north to find a caravan park for me and Caspers (his dog) to settle down in."

I simply said, "Oh, okay."

Yet, inside, I felt anxious about him travelling alone with a heart condition and sad that he wouldn't be around.

Situations that continued to trigger difficult emotions kept presenting themselves. For instance, although I had friends, they weren't in many of my classes that year. So, I had to ask if I could sit next to other students, which made me feel nervous, or else I sat alone and felt very self-conscious. Then, during lunchtime, my friends started playing handball with the boys, but I was too shy and embarrassed about how I looked and how bad I was at sports, so I didn't join in. Afterwards, I wrote in my journal that "I hate myself."

I also began hating myself for being irritable, angry and disrespectful at Mum's, while at Dad's, I kept smiling despite the pain within. Meanwhile, the low-grade depression I had since childhood was subtly growing. Fed up, I decided to do something about it.

The Diet

In fourth grade, I had learned I could achieve anything I put my mind to. So, I set goals again. This time, they weren't limited to good grades. I set goals in several areas of my life, my weight being one of them. Although I naturally started slimming out that year, I believed I would look better if I lost *just a little more weight*. From a lady who promoted dieting on a midday television show, I learnt to swap foods with higher fat content for those with less. I traded my breakfast of crumpets with butter and honey and my hot chocolate for Weet-Bix with light milk. Biscuit snacks were swapped for fruit and so on. I also started walking home from school.

The end of the year came, and I concluded that I had achieved none of my goals—a harsh exaggeration. With low self-esteem and high standards, I was overly critical of myself. Yet, there was one goal I achieved with flying colours. I lost a significant amount of weight. Losing weight gave me a sense of accomplishment and helped me to feel good, even somewhat attractive. I liked fitting into tight jeans and wearing midriff tops. I liked having self-control and my preoccupation with avoiding food. I soon discovered that dieting also made me feel detached from the world and parts of myself. Feeling light-headed and too tired to feel anything other than hunger brought the sense of detachment, as did being diet and exercise focused. With all of this combined, the life I knew disappeared, and a new one with what *seemed* like freedom and empowerment opened up.

3. Dusk

With my dieting continuing and anorexia developing, the summer holidays now revolved around avoiding food and excessively exercising. I recall Dad taking his wife, my little sister and me to McDonald's. Usually, my stepmother would order for us, but not this time. After mentally calculating which food had the least fat, I politely asked, "Is it okay if I order my food?" I had a small juice and half of my junior burger and fries, hoping not to draw attention to my dieting.

At Mum's, dinner was the only meal we ate together. Mum always allowed me to choose, to a degree, what I ate, so now I opted for dishes like steamed fish and vegetables instead of crumbed fish and chips. I dramatically cut back my eating at breakfast, lunch and snack times. Our new pup, Winnie, got many walks. And I secretly began exercising in our bathroom after showering.

I didn't dare tell anyone I wanted to lose weight or how I hated myself. I didn't feel these were things I could talk about. I felt embarrassed about my body and ashamed of how I acted at times, so I didn't want to draw attention to or connect with the "ugly" parts of myself by speaking about them. Having experienced unhelpful comments about my appearance and unwanted medical interventions as a child, I also felt guarded. I didn't want people speculating about my body. It was private. Nor did I want to alarm my parents and for them to monitor everything I was eating or try to stop my dieting and exercising. And even though I didn't talk about my dieting, Mum and Dad could see I was losing weight and wasn't myself.

I started tenth grade with little energy and fell asleep during classes. Along with my weight and energy decreasing, so did my interest in movie stars, who's dating who, talking during lessons and fashion, all the "normal" teenage things. I well and truly needed help by now. My friend Julie wrote me a letter. In the letter, Julie said she noticed I hadn't been myself and asked, "What's up?" I appreciated her care. Both my science and sports teachers expressed concern about my weight loss. I felt scared they would tell my parents they were concerned, yet relieved to have some people notice everything wasn't okay for me. The teachers, however, didn't intervene, but Mum did. Mum noticed the warning signs—weight loss, food preoccupation, over-exercising, withdrawal, eating less and mood changes, so she took me to see our family doctor. I was sure I was only dieting and didn't have anorexia. I certainly wasn't expecting to be referred to a dietitian and psychologist at an outpatient clinic for eating disorders.

The outpatient team talked about admitting me to an inpatient eating disorder program. My weight was now critically low and my period had stopped. I met the criteria for hospitalisation, but no beds were available, so they gave me extra time to gain weight at home. I felt shocked they were considering hospitalisation. I thought, *Sure, I'm thin and finding it hard to eat more and exercise less. Perhaps it's a problem, but it's no big deal.* With being so tired, food-focused and driven, along with liking being thin and disconnecting from the world, I felt no desire to change. I was crossing over from "normality" into anorexia in a numb state, not comprehending nor caring what I was stepping into.

My sense of urgency, however, arose when I sat down to a dinner Mum cooked, and I froze. I just stared at the plate. Although famished, I couldn't eat the meal, not even one vegetable. My mind was full of negative thoughts about myself and food, compounded by the effects of malnourishment, depression and perhaps even genetics; I lost all reason and ability to eat. I felt scared and trapped. My diet was no longer just a diet but a multi-layered disorder. I asked Mum if I could go to hospital sooner rather than later.

Inpatient Treatment

Two weeks later, they admitted me to an inpatient program for eating disorders. On arrival, I sat on my bed and stared downward at the grey and white speckled carpet. After what seemed like forever, they delivered my lunch. It was a buttered turkey sandwich and a small orange juice. I ate it and drank the juice. I was hungry. It was a reasonably sized lunch, and after all, I was there to get better. Then, the other eating disorder patients walked into our four bedded room. One girl stood as she ate and another played with her food. No one talked and no one completed their meal. There was one male patient with anorexia, but he was in the room next door with general patients. No nurse was appointed to bring encouragement at mealtimes or to document what was eaten. The girl standing as she ate had a tube going into her nose. *Gee, she must be really sick,* I thought. *Clearly, I'm a fake and shouldn't be here.* Instantly, self-criticism rather than hope reappeared, and so did rules about how much and what I could eat once again.

In the afternoon, I met with the doctor.

"Your BMI (body mass index) needs to be 18 before discharge. Does that freak you out?"

"No," I replied and meant it.

My BMI was above 18 before dieting, so I figured I would be happy to have a BMI of 18; but no more. I now faced a balancing act. I wanted to eat more and re-introduce different food types, but I didn't want to get too comfortable with eating that my weight would go above the "magic" BMI number. So, I calculated the fat and calorie content of everything I ate and watched the scales even more closely now.

I soon learnt the program had a three-tiered approach to treatment to help medically stabilise patients and provide an incentive to gain weight. So, most times, if we gained one kilo over the week, we could increase our gym activity and go home for a day or two. If we lost weight or didn't gain the kilo, we had to stay on our bed apart from toilet privileges, and leave wasn't allowed. If there was no improvement the next week, we had to be on strict bed rest. Strict bed rest was the worst. It meant using a bedpan, having a sponge wash and going to the hospital classroom on our bed. Leave or participation at the gym was certainly not permitted. Then, at any stage, if we were medically compromised or not progressing, the eating disorder team would consider inserting a nasal gastric (NG) tube. With an NG tube, which went up the nose and into the stomach, nurses could administer high-calorie supplements through the night.

Having "privileges" taken away, however, was not always helpful. I felt humiliated and degraded having to use a bedpan (although I was well enough to walk to the toilet) with just the privacy of a curtain around my bed, especially while teenage boys were visiting other patients in the room. I had an NG tube inserted, a painful procedure that added to my humiliation. I hated my family and friends seeing me with it. I believed it conveyed the message that I wasn't eating at all, which was untrue. Then, at times, I felt so depressed that the program provided no incentive to eat and gain weight. Nevertheless, it did stabilise my physical health, which was important, though a more holistic and tailor-made approach may have been helpful.

I voiced my frustrations with treatment, as most fifteen-year-olds would, only to hear staff say, "It's just the eating disorder talking," or "This is fantastic; she is now feeling anger and can express herself." Not only did I feel oppressed having to comply with aspects of a program I disagreed with, but I also felt my voice, thoughts and feelings were discounted.

Unlike most teenagers, though, my life now consisted of being woken three times a week for 6 am weigh-ins. I had to use a bedpan, put on a hospital gown and step onto scales. Next, they served breakfast by my bedside. I could select what food to order as long as it was on my meal plan devised by the dietitian. I then walked to the hospital classroom for schooling until lunchtime. Like the rest of the meals and snacks, lunch was served by our bedsides. After lunch and half an hour of bed rest, I had to attend craft sessions or meet with the dietitian. I wasn't allowed to see a psychologist at this point. They explained it would be of little benefit to talk with someone when so undernourished (I disagreed). I did, however, join in a couple of family therapy sessions. From these, I received the impression that the team believed my anorexia stemmed from my mum's eating disorder. It felt like they didn't acknowledge that I was my own person with my own struggles.

Two months passed, and despite some weight gain, I was still very underweight. Self-criticism, lies, starvation and fear shaped my thoughts and feelings. With little energy and a lot of anxiety, I couldn't think clearly and devised more rules and routines to follow. I became focused on details and unable to see the "big picture." I could no longer concentrate on schoolwork or absorb what people were saying. Beliefs founded on lies played over and over in my mind. Spontaneity, living in the moment and connecting with my heart now felt scary.

Food obsession went hand in hand with starvation. Looking up and memorising the fat and calorie content of food and drinks became my new and sole hobby. I felt drawn to magazines and television programs that featured recipes and dreamt of food. I constantly thought about the next meal and calculated everything I ate. It took hours to work out what I could allow myself to eat. Still, I never felt at ease with the permission I gave myself, so OCD would take over. Numbers and orders, rules and routines dictated what I could and couldn't eat and do, and somehow—my free will seemingly ceased to exist.

Yet, an element of anorexia enticed me. It was comforting to have a food obsession, something to occupy my mind with, rather than feeling empty or distressed. Unable to speak about my innermost feelings, anorexia gave me a voice, expressing through my weight that all was not well. Rules and routines helped me to get through each day despite depression and enabled me to control my intake and weight. Fading away even brought a level of freedom from self-consciousness and social anxiety. Moreover, punishing myself through deprivation and pushing myself to achieve strangely felt good, relieving and even spiritual. It was as though I was getting rid of the "bad" parts of myself that I hated.

Inpatient treatment, although testing, also had its appeal. I liked escaping from the life I had lost interest in. I liked forming friendships with other eating disordered patients who I related to. I liked the distraction that craft groups provided. I especially liked breathing in fresh air, feeling the warmth of the sun and glimpsing natural light as we walked through the courtyard to the next building for physio, something I previously took for granted. I also liked physio itself. I learnt how to properly stretch and lift weights; helping me to feel centred and physically good. Above all, I secretly liked how the program permitted me to eat more and varied foods. Allowing some "forbidden" foods, which tasted incredibly good in light of starvation, provided something to look forward to each day. Although I would never admit it aloud food had become my life source, what I was living and almost dying for.

Having almost reached my goal weight after thirteen weeks of hospitalisation, I didn't think I looked fat, yet I felt unbearably big. Fidgeting on bed rest, all I could think was, *I want to get out of this body.* Being extremely underweight all year, my body, although still very thin, in comparison now felt large. And even though outwardly I was recovering, inwardly, nothing had changed, leaving me feeling distressed and stuck in a body that I didn't identify with. I wasn't ready or equipped to deal with the weight gain. Yet, as I had been an inpatient for so long and was medically stable, the team decided it was time for discharge.

At home, I focused on maintaining weight, returning to school and achieving goals. A few weeks later, I had a follow-up appointment as an outpatient. Not meaning to, I had lost weight. I needed better support. Being given a goal weight less than my set-point weight also didn't help. Against my wishes, they re-admitted me to hospital.

The doctor said, "If you don't make progress, we'll have to transfer you to the adolescent psychiatric unit." That was meant to be an incentive for me to progress. I didn't. I was transferred.

Adolescent Psych Unit

I instantly took a dislike to the adolescent psych unit. I felt treated like a child. A nurse met with me and the other patients each morning to plan the day together, from the moment we woke until we went to sleep. I had to adhere to strict rules and was constantly under watch. The only good part was being allowed home on weekends. On my first weekend home, desperate not to return to the unit, I drank a large amount of water to the point of throwing up. It worked. The staff believed I was sick and allowed me to stay home a couple of days longer. The following weekend, I felt compelled to eat out-of-date food to make myself sick again and get out of treatment. It didn't work. I had no choice but to return to the unit.

The adolescent unit was where teenagers with behavioural issues and mental illnesses were monitored and supported. Six of us stayed there overnight, Monday to Friday. Throughout the day, fifteen or so teenagers attended the school there too. Along with following their general rules and attending school, I had to have bed rest after each meal, supervision at mealtimes and be wheelchaired around the grounds if I lost weight. Despite hating the restrictions, I discovered this place wasn't that bad. There were only a couple of us there with anorexia, and there was a lot of focus on schooling and partaking in activities like snooker and video games. Most of the staff, teachers included, were caring and supportive too. Such an environment allowed the eating disorder world to become less and for me to eat a little more and maintain a semi-safe but low weight.

They allowed me to attend my high school twice a week. Attending equated to wagging. I thought, *Why sit at a desk when I could walk?* I walked for hours on end. I felt compelled. To stop would mean standing up against anorexia, and I wasn't ready for that. I got away with truancy for a while. The staff at the adolescent unit thought I was at school, and the teachers at school thought I was at the unit. Somehow, someone found out what was happening, and I had to sign in at the principal's office each morning before school. Yet, it didn't stop me from skipping classes to walk.

On weekends, rain, hail or shine, I also had to walk. On a cold winter day, I layered up my clothes, put on my beanie and heated a wheat pack to hold against my body as I prepared to head out. Then, walking down the street, a car pulled over, and anxiety rushed over me.

"Cas, do you want a lift?" asked my friend's dad, who I barely knew.

"No, thank you, I enjoy walking," I lied.

"But it's raining. I'll drive you home."

"Maybe next time, I'm fine, but thank you," I lied again.

I wasn't walking for enjoyment, I wasn't okay and I had no intention of receiving a lift in the future. I walked a few blocks before a different car pulled over, and another concerned parent offered me a ride. It happened regularly, so I took to walking back streets. Twice, men followed me, undoubtedly with bad intentions. Fortunately, I could make it to safety. Although the incidents scared me, I still walked the backstreets, avoiding people who knew me.

Back at the unit, I had to attend school. I certainly couldn't wag it and go for walks. Each class had around five students ranging between the ages of twelve to eighteen years old. Most students came for schooling and counselling and went home afterwards. We studied for half the day, and the other half, we did art or played sports. Never had I liked playing sports until now. A typical basketball game isn't so typical when the teams consist of young people struggling with issues ranging from OCD, drug addiction, attention deficit disorder and bipolar. I loved it! Everyone encouraged and accepted one another and pulled each other into line when needed. Watching people accommodate each other's particularities in the game was also pretty amusing. For example, some had to bounce the ball a certain number of times, while others dodged the ball altogether. Hanging out together worked well for sports, but having group therapy once or twice a week was hopeless. Interesting, for sure, but not beneficial.

I also saw a couple of psychologists at the unit. They were caring but of little help. One focused on family therapy. She discussed how I could be a better daughter and help Mum more around the house. It was a nice idea but a complete waste of time, not to mention it fuelled my belief that I was a bad daughter.

My nurse, Lexi, also asked, "Are you not concerned about what you are doing to your body and that you may be unable to have children one day?" I could see she was trying to help, even though she said it in a frustrated and almost blaming manner, but it was unhelpful. I was locked in a complex disorder—anorexia was not a lifestyle choice. I needed a radical inner change to take place so that I could even contemplate recovery. Thinking about my body and future children certainly wouldn't suffice.

Still, I hadn't lost hope of finding a way forward. During bed rest, I read classic self-help books like *Feel the Fear and Do It Anyway* by Susan Jeffers[1] and *Chicken Soup for the Soul* by Jack Canfield and Mark V. Hansen.[2] I soaked in the many letters that Tanya, Dianna and other school friends had written, and meditated on poetry that explored faith, hope and love. I still believed God was probably real and life had purpose and meaning, but I didn't know what that looked like. In a way, anorexia gave me a pause button on day-to-day life and provided space to dig deep. And while I wasn't intentionally searching out God, my soul longed for something more, and I continued to read and ponder. Unknowingly, I was spiritually hungry.

Remaining underweight, but with the summer holidays approaching and the unit closing, I was discharged and referred to a psychologist and dietitian in my hometown. They were kind yet counterproductive. The psychologist wanted me to role-play with dolls to help express what I was feeling. I thought, *Are you serious? I'm almost seventeen years old!* While the dietitian devised a meal plan for me that was nearly as restrictive as my eating disorder. Perhaps if I had spoken with professionals who specialised in eating disorders, I may have felt better supported and safe.[3]

Soon, Christmas Day arrived. My family tried to make it enjoyable, but it wasn't. I had taken my own food to my grandparents, and I felt guilty about turning down theirs. I wanted to please them, but I couldn't. I loved roast dinners and wanted to eat the lunch Gran had cooked, but again, with anorexia, I couldn't. A once joyful and anticipated event had become overshadowed by anxiety and shame.

In the new year, I returned to the adolescent unit. My treatment team set weight goals for me, told me I needed to eat all the food on my meal plan and talked about homelife, school and my thoughts about weight gain. We never touched on anything deep. They didn't see that underneath anorexia, an inner journey of searching out and discerning what was important to me was taking place.

My relationship with Dad was one area of my life that I knew was important and worth investing in. So, I signed us up for the local bushwalkers club, where we went on treks through the mountains and along the coastal line during weekend leave. I loved being outdoors with Dad and collecting wildflowers on the trails. It involved exercise, the reason I "had" to choose this activity over watching movies or going for car drives and picnics, but it also had healthy and healing aspects.

I invited Dad to Thursday baking nights at the adolescent unit. In typical Dad style, he always added "just a bit extra" or "a secret ingredient" to our cakes and slices, so fun and mess was always the final product. Although I never ate the baking, it was good for me (and Dad, I suspect) to share special one-on-one father and daughter times. I guess we did our own family therapy.

Along with spending time with Dad, forming friendships at the unit was also therapeutic. Standing in an empty classroom, a male friend confided, "I'm crazy. At least what you do makes sense."

"I know I'm skinny, but I can't even let myself eat an apple when I feel hungry. Now that's crazy!" came my honest reply.

Tom, a fourteen-year-old boy, said loudly as he entered the communal dining room, "Cas, you're scaring me now. You're looking too thin."

And yet another, "I feel for you, eating your food like a little bird."

These guys were dealing with their issues, yet had the compassion to reach out and support me and other patients. When I was on bed rest, three boys took turns sitting by my door to keep me company and cheer me up. Like big brothers looking out for their sister, they also stood up for me and told the staff that my restrictions (i.e., not being allowed to use the phone as I hadn't gained weight) were unfair.

Feeling encouraged and accepted, my anxiety around boys even dropped to where, one afternoon, I casually wore a green facial mask while playing a board game with them. I joined the boys in snooker and video games, too, which I was hopeless at but I didn't care. Forming friendships with the guys provided teenage normality, not to mention a good distraction from the disorder and surroundings, which was helpful in itself.

Making friends at the unit, however, also meant hearing stories of tremendous pain, abuse and trauma. One girl, Maggie, disclosed, "I'm in and out of institutions so much that I don't remember people's names, so I swap something of mine with something of theirs to remember them by." She swapped me her green silk tie. Tragically, Maggie only lived another year before taking her own life. Another girl, Lien, suffered trauma as a refugee, yet she took the time to create a gift during craft and handed it to me with a big, gentle smile. These new friends showed me a different side to life. Their resilience, strength and genuine kindness were admirable. And although outwardly nothing changed, inwardly, I was certainly learning and growing along the way.

Different Approaches

I maintained a low weight but made no further progress, so they transferred me back to the inpatient eating disorder program. During a visit, Dad took me outside to the balcony and encouraged me to yell, "Anorexia, go away!" I spoke it aloud. I didn't yell it. I wasn't ready for it to go away. I also didn't believe it would help. Looking back, however, it was pretty cool Dad took that approach—there is power in the spoken word.

Several weeks passed, and I barely gained weight, so they discharged me. Within weeks of being at home, Dad heard how I had lost more weight and drove to Mum's to pick me up and take me back to the hospital. He literally picked me up as I refused to go. I always tried my best to please Dad, but this time I couldn't. I believed being in treatment was going to make matters worse. Reluctantly, he carried me to the car and drove me to the hospital. I understood he was acting out of care and responsibility.

My school friends hadn't given up on me either. On my seventeenth birthday, they chipped in for concert tickets to see *Bon Jovi* live in the city. I was allowed to leave the hospital for the day and snuck back into my room late at night. There was a part of me that was still like any other teenager. That was a good birthday.

Following this, the team took a novel approach to treatment. It involved inserting an NG tube down each of us with anorexia and administering a supplement through the tube, called TwoCal. The aim was to get us all to the same weight. They explained, "You are all around the same age and height, and once you reach the weight target, the tube can come out, and you can relearn to eat." We were also told, "It would be good if you can eat between supplements, but you don't have to." I was starving and relied on the push to gain weight each week to allow myself to eat, but now I had no reason to. I knew depression would set in without my food preoccupation. So, I ate a hundred per cent normally while on supplements, partly in rebellion, mostly in survival mode from depression. I felt sick and had awful stomach cramps. I curled up on my bed with a heat pack to ease the pain. Late one afternoon, I was so full that I threw up while the nurse was syringing the supplement down my tube. I felt frightened as the NG tube that went up my nose, down my throat to my stomach, came out of my mouth. The nurse looked stunned and sought advice before removing the tube, inserting a new one and re-administering the TwoCal. After I gained seven kilos in one week (the aim was one to two kilos per week) and my legs swelled with fluid retention, the eating disorder team cut back the supplements, and I returned to restricting my intake, as I had planned.

One of the parents of another girl with anorexia commented, "Gee, you've gained a lot of weight in a short time," which I knew and didn't need reminding of. After the weight gain, I made no further progress and once again was discharged.

Unintentionally, I lost weight at home and was re-admitted to the same program. Fed up with treatment and feeling hopeless, I overdosed on paracetamol. I didn't want to die. I just desperately wanted the team to see how unhappy I was. I sat on my bed and didn't even join the exercise groups. The nurse unit manager tried his best to encourage me to go for supervised walks with the other patients, saying, "You don't want to end up fat like me." He didn't offend me. I knew he was joking and cared.

To be fair, although treatment was ineffective for me, the eating disorder team, which included doctors, nurses, psychologists, dietitians and physios, were genuinely caring. The hospital schoolteachers, craft lady and most of the general nurses were also kind and supportive. And in time, they arranged a dining table in the communal room for supervised meals. Dietetic groups began, and they allowed me to see a psychologist.

The team even organised a couple of day trips. One was to a theme park, the other to a country homestead for horse riding. The outings meant more exercise and provoked anxiety about eating lunch out, so they weren't fun-filled events, but they were still a refreshing change from the treatment setting.

We also had two ladies from a popular teen magazine visit the ward to discuss body image and the influence media has on young people. I loved reading girly magazines with my friends in the schoolyard, especially the health, relationship and body sections. I felt drawn to dieting, fitness and beauty articles for self-improvement advice. And while I paid little attention to the models, it was eye-opening to learn that day how they photoshopped all the images of the models, which made me realise that *Even they aren't as perfect as they seem.*

Nevertheless, I didn't progress, and they discharged me. The doctor said, "You look fine, so we are letting you go home." With a BMI of less than 18, I certainly didn't look or feel fine. Instead, I looked a bit healthier than I did on admission. Mum was in a psychiatric unit in our hometown, so they discharged me to Dad's.

Dad adopted a proactive role in trying to help me eat. He arranged for his wife to serve me small meals at their kitchen table and said, "If you're eating, we can go for walks together." Yet, I didn't eat small portions of everyday foods. I ate small to medium portions of specific diet foods in specific ways and after completing specific tasks. I also ate for comfort and reward, so having a meal set before me with the rest of the family was difficult, near impossible, to eat. I felt anxious at mealtimes and embarrassed about my eating habits. I knew I was overly fussy with my food and not setting a good example for my little sister. Dad also tried to hide my exercise weights and glued together pages in a magazine, which I assume featured diets. I guess he tried to set up a home program for me. Yet, despite my family doing their best to help, with depression growing and wanting to avoid feeling hunger pains, I just slept the days away.

Not surprisingly, I was re-admitted to inpatient treatment. I spent Christmas Eve being cannulated and hooked up to intravenous (IV) fluids as my temperature read below 36°C. In the morning, the nurse found the thermometer was faulty, so the IV fluids ceased, and they gave me leave for Christmas lunch with Mum. We had a quiet picnic at the park, where I stuck with eating "safe" foods (foods that didn't threaten anorexia), helping to keep my anxiety at bay and making the outing somewhat enjoyable.

Mum and I returned to the hospital half an hour late only to be greeted with, "You're late, and it's going to be recorded," by the nurse in charge.

Mum also overheard another nurse call me a "twit" and confronted her. Although only a few nurses were unkind, their demeanour influenced the atmosphere and left me feeling angry and alone.

On top of this, the eating disorder program had also stopped during Christmas time. There was no one else but me on the ward with anorexia, and no groups or classes were running. So, I sat on my bed all day and felt it didn't matter whether I ate, or not. The program at least permitted me to eat a bit more. It also let me fill my head all day with precise food, weight and exercise calculations and allowed me to stick to routines and complete tasks to allow myself to eat. Now, with no incentive to eat, I froze. I lost all reason to eat all over again. Depressed, I cried uncontrollably for hours on end. I felt no life within or around me. I felt nothing. It was like I was dead but stuck in my body alive. I had a disturbing daydream of hanging myself, and each step was strangely and darkly comforting, in every way.

My only relief was to sneak off the ward and go for long walks or catch a train to the nearby mall. My non-compliance ended up with me having a public guardian to keep me safe and to reinforce compliance with treatment, treatment that barely existed.

As nothing seemed to help, they referred me to one of Australia's leading experts in eating disorders. Mum and I met with the psychiatrist in his large city office. His manner was gentle, and he had a thorough understanding of anorexia. After considering our circumstances, he arranged for us to try inpatient treatment—together.

N.B. A gentle reminder. If you find my story challenging, please reach out to someone for support. And check out the *Resource* section at the back for information on seeking support and implementing self-help.

4. A Long Night

On the 18th of January 1999, Mum and I were both admitted to a private psych hospital. Besides its old, musty smell, it seemed more homely than the other facilities. It also offered a well-structured eating disorder program with group sessions, meal support and high expectations of normalising eating and weight. It was a full on, strict program. At this point, I needed a more simplified individual treatment plan, one that also gently explored spirituality. Overtaken by anorexia, however, I couldn't express what I needed. Instead, outward signs of rebellion and eating disorder behaviours spoke for me.

As Mum was doing much better than I, a nurse remarked in front of other patients, "Look what you are doing to your mother. You are making her suffer. You're not behaving like a Christian."

I hated that. Anorexia was tormenting enough. I didn't need judgements and misguided corrections too. I was losing all sense of self, and having people only see and correct the eating disorder—rather than see and affirm me as a person—made me drift even further away.

Hate and anger now took turns with depression. I hated sitting with other people at the dining table. I hated having no choice about what food I could eat and the rules and supervision around food. I hated that there were particular foods I let myself eat, but the program did not. I hated being assigned a special room behind the nurses' desk, where they could keep an eye on me through a window. I hated the therapy groups and having to sit down in them. This treatment would have been helpful at the start, but now it only felt suffocating and way beyond where I was at.

To top it off, I lost weight, and the doctor said I needed a percutaneous endoscopic gastrostomy (PEG) tube inserted into my stomach for supplements. I had pulled out multiple NG tubes, so they opted for this tube instead, which I couldn't pull out. On hearing this, I felt trapped. I relied on weight gain targets to allow myself to eat. Now that tube feeding would gain weight for me, and more rapidly than my mind and emotions could deal with, I felt no permission to eat. This equated to major depression, and I couldn't handle that. I told the head doctor to "f--- off" as I pushed over the blood pressure device and stormed out of the room. They needed me to fast before the procedure, so I headed straight for the fruit bowl in the dining room, grabbed a pear and took a bite while hurrying down the driveway and out of the hospital grounds. A nurse ran after me, grabbed the fruit from my hand, and escorted me back to my room. After many tears, they transported me to day surgery to have the PEG tube inserted. The tube was often infected, much bigger than I expected and left a scar. It was uncomfortable and unpleasant. Any inspiration within me to go forward was now gone.

Adult Psych Unit

In a matter of days, they transferred me to yet another hospital. My nurse assured me I would only be there overnight for medical observation. When the morning came, however, at just seventeen years old, they moved me to a general adult psychiatric unit. I stood in denial as the doctor said, "You'll be staying here for four weeks, so you can be near the hospital in case you need medical attention. Afterwards, you can resume treatment with your mother."

"Do you mind sitting down to fill out your admission form?" asked the nurse.

"I'm not sitting or filling out any form," I bluntly replied.

I felt scared and angered at being there. That night, I went to bed not knowing the unit's location. I had no mobile phone and no contact with any familiar faces.

Sal, the patient in the room next door, woke me in the morning. Sal was a cross-dresser who lived with paraplegia. He was yelling and swearing at the nurses, "Get me the f---- up," so he could have an early coffee. Molly, an elderly lady in the neighbouring room, mimicked Sal's every word. When the nurses didn't come to help Sal, he threw his urinal bottle into the corridor, causing blood and urine to spill past my doorway. Distressed and enraged, Sal then dragged himself across the floor, out of his room and towards the nurse's station. It felt overwhelming, to say the least, awakening to adults who were extremely mentally and emotionally unwell.

I then met Nurse Jaine. She informed me I needed to come to the dining room for each meal, where I could choose food from the servery per my meal plan. Nurses would supervise me during mealtimes, and I was not to "play" with my food, or else they would throw it out. I was to stay in my room, in my pyjamas and rest until 2 pm each day, apart from meals and supervised toileting. Afterwards, I could shower, watch television, join therapy groups (none were running, as they were understaffed) and see my doctor and dietitian.

The program was basic, and I hated residing in my room until the afternoon. I disagreed with the reasoning behind it. I stood on the veranda before 2 pm one day, only to be told to go to my room. I grabbed the railing and pleaded, "Can't I just stand here for half an hour in the sunshine?" That didn't get me far. The nurse unclenched my hands and took me back to my room, where I stood in the freezing cold air-conditioning instead.

Like other programs, weigh-ins occurred at 6 am three times a week. I felt anxious as I waited for the nurse to weigh me. *What if I put on more weight than required? What if I lost weight? I should have eaten more. I should have eaten less. I should have drunk more water before being weighed*, and on and on, the thoughts circled. Upon finding out my weight, calculations replaced my anxiety. I calculated every calorie I consumed the previous week and made a mental list of what foods to eat and avoid in the coming one. Even if I gained the required weight, I had no peace of mind. I only ate part of the meal plan and over-exercised, so gaining the required amount meant halting any idea of increasing my intake and decreasing my exercise. The fact that I was starving, medically unstable and knew I looked extremely underweight made no difference to my response about my weight. It was all about numbers, orders and rules—countless rules.

Random room checks also occurred on the program, where nurses confiscated items like diet food, exercise equipment and calorie books to promote recovery. However, more often than not, how they conducted these made me feel manipulative, sneaky, naughty and unworthy. It was like I wasn't a real person but just an anorexic. Adding to this, some staff seemed to believe everything I said or did was eating disordered. One nurse, for instance, watched me pour a glass of water and said, "I know what you are doing," implying that I was engaging in an eating disorder behaviour. I explained, "I'm thirsty. I just want a drink." He laughed and shook his head. I don't think he understood how weak, vulnerable and tormented I already felt and how such comments made me further distressed and drained. What would have been more helpful is if he had asked why I was getting a drink and listened to my response, while considering my needs.

Nonetheless, there were kind staff, like the kitchen ladies, who smiled and asked, "How are you doing?" And well-meaning nurses who simply struggled to help us. One nurse removed our food trays at the start of each meal, not giving us time to eat or drink anything. All our food and drinks got tipped into the bin over the weekend, and she recorded that we refused to eat. She later apologised, saying, "Sorry, I don't know how to help you girls," and took a few days' leave after the incident. Another nurse thought I should eat cake instead of the fruit the dietitian had ordered, and she was frustrated when I refused to. She also apologised, confessing, "I don't know much about anorexia, but I'm learning."

Along with the challenges of treatment, the facility itself was unpleasant. The washing machine was often broken, so thoroughly exhausted, I hand-washed and hung out my clothes on the veranda, only to have items go missing. The dishwasher regularly broke too. So, we had to use plastic plates and cups. And on weekends, the unit ran out of linen and towels (so I quickly learnt to stash them on Fridays). Some general psych patients would even urinate in the corridors and walk around naked. The only place I could retreat to was a courtyard full of smokers, which smelt like a nauseating mix of coffee, urine, body odour and tobacco, all at once.

Insanity and brokenness were everywhere. I heard my nurse scream as a patient stabbed her in the neck with a knife (she survived). I also heard patients screaming outside my window as they arrived by police wagons during the night. Then, in the months to come, a lady with bipolar disorder bought me a blue and yellow flower before tragically hanging herself three rooms up from mine.

Severe Anorexia

I felt utterly exhausted, freezing, dizzy, angry, starving, obsessed, shut down, desperate and as though I was losing complete touch with reality.

My mind was plagued by not only critical thoughts but also condemning and tormenting ones too. I now fell into the severe to extreme category for anorexia.[4] I felt dominated by the disorder, detrimental treatment and unhealthy surroundings. It was relentless, with no respite.

Even so, some people said I had good self-control and wished they had the same level of control as me. Others made judgements and said I was selfish by having anorexia. Truth is—I felt controlled by an outer force and had no sense of self. I had to hide food in my pockets, sleeves, napkins, slits cut into my jacket and under my dinner plate whenever I could, even though I was starving, and it was highly anxiety-provoking. I relied solely on nurses watching, encouraging and recording my intake for me to eat. I couldn't sleep past 6 am and woke in fear during the night, unsure if it was okay to rest in bed. I could no longer entertain thoughts that opposed the eating disorder, and I most definitely could not voice them. It was like being trapped in an abusive relationship, just as Jenni Schaffer describes in her book *Life Without Ed*.[5] The eating disorder conditionally met some needs while eroding and denying any sense of self and basic freedoms.

With severe anorexia, even things that had nothing to do with food, weight or exercise were now forbidden. A young nurse discovered this whilst attempting to pop headphones onto my head, saying, "Here, listen to this music. I think you'll like it." Panicked, I could hardly breathe and shook my head. She insisted. I declined again. I believed in doing so, feelings would return to my heart. I'd eat more, gain weight, lose anorexia and be back to square one of being me and engulfed by emptiness. I feared that tremendously. The fear ran so deep into my very soul. I didn't just fear that "being me" would equate to being my natural weight and depressed with my appearance. I feared "being me" would leave me as a complete mess or depressed beyond measure, with all the inner ugliness of my sin and defectiveness rising and spilling over, with no way of controlling it. Interlinked with this, I further believed taking just one extra bite or enjoying something non-food related was declaring, "I am worthy, and life is worthwhile," but I was not convinced. I felt trapped—on every level, in every way.

N.B. I was worthy; we are all worthy,
and life is worthwhile. I just didn't know it yet.

It was now March, and after the four weeks were up, the doctor said, "You're still medically unstable and will be here longer than we planned."

"Really?" I felt numb. "When can I leave?"

"We can't give you a discharge date at this point."

The only immediate plan the eating disorder team had for me was sedation. Against my wishes, I had to swallow haloperidol, a strong antipsychotic drug known to have adverse side effects. Their reason for sedation was that I stood all day and paced the unit. I wasn't on anti-depressants or medication for anxiety, so I'm unsure why haloperidol was their first line of choice. After taking the drug, I wanted to cry but couldn't. I tried to exercise but couldn't. I felt weird and doped out. It felt awful. I was barely present within myself amidst anorexia, and now I was grasping to have any hold at all on being present. Haloperidol affected me more than I could cope with. I had also been in treatment for months on end without leave, and I thought I'd go crazy unless I got out.

I had a plan. I'd ask a nurse who didn't know my strict program for my bank card and money, which they kept in a locked drawer. I'd then casually walk out of the unit via the courtyard when they were performing hourly checks on patients. It worked. I found myself on a busy road and hopped on a crowded bus, not knowing where it was going. Lucky for me, it drove straight to the train station. I found a phone booth and quickly flicked through my little phone book. The only person my parents didn't know very well or where they lived was a guy I made friends with at the adolescent psych unit (who I had a crush on). I called his number and spoke with his sister. I told her I was friends with her brother and asked if I could stay with them for a few days. Her family, not fully knowing how unwell I was, kindly said, "Yes."

My friend's father met me at another train station and drove me to their home. There, I phoned Mum, "I'm safe. I'm at a friend's place. I need time out, but I'll return soon." In the meantime, my school friends searched for me, and police officers questioned them about where I might be and searched my home. Somehow, the situation escalated, and my absconding was even aired on television. Unbeknownst to me, I also featured on the front page of several newspapers, making my private struggle very public. After the guy's parents, who I was staying with, saw the television reports, they promptly drove me back to the private psych hospital Mum was at. I hoped to stay there with her. Instead, I got an ambulance ride with a police escort back to the adult psych unit.

Once at the unit, they told me how silly I was for running away and said, "Don't you know how sick you are?" I knew I was extremely unwell, but it made no difference. I just needed to get out of that place. While out, I also cut the PEG tube, hoping it wouldn't work and they'd remove it. I thought without having supplements, I'd be able to allow myself to eat more. However, they saw the cut tube as a sign that I ran away because I feared weight gain. I explained myself, but no one listened. Instead, I had to lay on my bed while they removed the PEG tube and replaced it with a new one. I felt a sharp burning pain in my stomach and saw blood spurt from the incision onto the wall. Yet, no kind words of reassurance were spoken.

To make sure I wouldn't run away again, I was specialled. Being specialled, much to my dislike, entailed having a nurse within one metre from me, day and night, everywhere I went, shower and toilet included. They also scheduled me. Being scheduled meant they could enforce treatment against my parents and my own wishes. At least they didn't put me back on haloperidol, which was a relief.

Still, I felt compelled and anxious to get out of the unit any chance I could. I pleaded with the eating disorder team, "Can I please attend the hospital chapel on Sunday? I'll return straight away."

"No, you haven't earned that privilege," was the resounding reply.

They did, however, arrange for the chaplain to visit. The chaplain had poor insight into anorexia and had nothing deeply inspiring to share, but I valued her caring presence, nonetheless. During this time, I also had a surprise visit from the youth group of Foothills Church, the church I started casually attending the previous year. I felt embarrassed that I looked so thin and had a nurse sitting beside me, but I was impressed that they travelled by train for over an hour to see me. Paul, the pastor of the church, also kept in contact. He sent me a letter from Indonesia, where he was ministering at the time. Within the letter, he shared Psalm 121:1-8:

"I lift up my eyes to the mountains—where does my help come from? My help comes from the Lord, the Maker of heaven and earth. He will not let your foot slip—he who watches over you will not slumber. He will watch over your life; the Lord will watch over your coming and going both now and forevermore." New International Version (NIV)

On a rare occasion, they granted me leave for a few hours. It was for Tanya's eighteenth birthday. I'm sure there were far more exciting things she could have done to celebrate her birthday rather than travelling to a psych unit to hang out with me, but she is an exceptional friend. We always celebrated birthdays together, and this one wouldn't be any different. I couldn't eat cake, drink wine or enjoy lunch at a café. So, we walked to the nearby mall, bought a packet of cigars and some scratchies and hopped into a photo booth to mark the occasion.

Three days later, it was my eighteenth, and for the first time in almost a year, I was allowed home for the weekend. Entering my house felt strange. It was like walking into the past while feeling detached from my surroundings all at once. Later that night, Dad came over, and we drove to a bar for a small celebration drink. Afterwards, Mum and I had photos taken together. The prints remain hidden in my bedroom closet. I looked dreadful, not just skeletal, but like I had been homeless for years and about to die. Returning to the adult psych unit, Nurse Jaine eyed me up and down before saying, "Come with me. I want to weigh you." Sure enough, I had lost weight, and they promptly inserted an NG tube. I was then moved to the locked ward, where I couldn't escape—not the best start to adulthood.

The locked ward held a few adults with severe psychiatric illnesses who required close monitoring due to being considered a danger to themselves and/or others. My nurse showed me my room. It had a small window the nurses could peep through at any time. Outside my room were a couple of dining tables, a phone and a television. There was also an enclosed veranda, which looked more like a prison with its wire fence. The other patients were too unwell to talk with, and the nurses sat hidden in their office. Apart from containing me and making me feel unsafe, the locked ward didn't achieve much. I walked around the small room for hours on end and missed out on meals because there was no eating disorder program there.

Despite it being unhelpful, I found myself in the locked ward again. The team moved me there because they wanted to separate me and another patient with anorexia. They said we were a bad influence on each other.

Admittedly, we sneaked Diet Coke from the vending machine together and hid sugar-free lollies in places where the nurses wouldn't look, like in the puzzle boxes in the communal lounge room. Yet, considering how unwell we were, these "behaviours" were relatively trivial in the grand scheme of things. I felt scared and angered. It seemed an overreaction to place me in the locked ward for this.

At another point, they put me in the seclusion room, which had padded walls and only a bare mattress on the floor. Nurse Jaine explained, "We're putting you here to help you. You need to calm down, your crying is disturbing the other patients." I eventually stopped crying, worn out, but again, nothing was accomplished through this tactic—besides feeling uncared for.

Along with mentally and emotionally struggling, I was extremely physically unwell too. I had muscle wastage in my legs. I had to lift my legs with my hands to get out of bed. I couldn't easily walk up steps, and if they were large steps, I couldn't walk up them at all. Being so underweight, even the blankets at night felt heavy, and I started getting sores on my hip bones from my jeans rubbing against them.

My digestive system was also compromised. I told the eating disorder team several times that I felt constipated. I could hardly walk or stand straight because of the pain. They didn't listen. My nurse did, however, open the toilet door without knocking. She saw me bent over, holding my stomach, accused me of throwing up and reported it to the team. Distressed and with little energy, I explained, "I wasn't vomiting. I was holding my stomach in pain with the constipation." Although they knew I didn't have bulimia and that constipation is a common side effect of anorexia, they dismissed what I said. It wasn't until I couldn't keep down water at the dining table (because I was so blocked up) that they decided I needed medication for my bowels. Not only did I need laxatives, but I also had to fast, stay on bed rest, have a drip and be closely monitored because I wasn't treated soon enough. Instead of receiving an apology, the doctor, behind closed doors said, "You did this to yourself."

Life was far gone, and so was I. I had anger, sadness, and food and exercise rules, which no one could interfere with. I feared nothing, apart from connecting with my heart and letting anorexia go. I knew precisely how to maximise my exercise and minimise my intake and broke every treatment rule to do so. I frequently escaped from the unit even though I was under close watch. I continued to resist treatment that I thought was unfair, and one time, I even had two male nurses restrain me to ensure compliance. I no longer cared what anyone thought. I was known as "the negotiator," and staff were cautioned not to listen to me. Mum said she no longer knew who I was. I was much like the heroin addict played by Leo DiCaprio in the movie *The Basketball Diaries*.

I looked like an addict too. My eyes were dull with dark rings, my olive complexion had turned pale and my teeth were discoloured. My hair was also long, thin and split, as I wouldn't sit to have it cut. I had lost all interest in dressing nicely, and with feeling cold all the time, my wardrobe consisted of oversized black coats, beanies and scarves. Painting my nails, applying makeup, fashion accessories or perfume didn't even cross my mind.

When gifted flowers or cards, instead of enjoying them like I used to, I didn't even look at them. They went into my cupboard straight away. Anorexia no longer allowed me to feel or relate to anything outside the disorder. There was no reasoning behind my response anymore. It was simply an automatic, *I must get rid of it. I can't stand it,* reaction. To even still myself for a moment to challenge my thoughts and behaviours was out of the question. Anything good breaking into my world, I instantly rejected—including the love of my family and friends. Mum experienced this when she walked into the unit one day for a visit while holding a pot plant, and I pleaded from a distance rather loudly, "Go away." I also turned down visits from friends. I wasn't angry or upset with my mum or friends, nor did I want to hurt them. I turned down visits as anorexia ruled every moment of every day. Compulsions had replaced reasoning. Bad had become good; good had become bad. And love on any level, I would not let touch me.

Beautiful Light

As the year progressed, once again, I didn't. I found myself at the same weight as on admission and in the same, if not worse, state of mind. Yet, since I had spent so much time in treatment with barely any leave, they allowed me to go home for the weekend. At home, as night fell, I curled up on my cold, hard, wooden bedroom floor in deep depression. Out of nowhere, peace, like an energy-filled light, swept through me over and over again. I don't recall praying and asking God for peace, but by his love, power and wisdom, he intervened at just the right time—bringing light amidst the darkness. Remarkably, the peace didn't scare or repel me. It perfectly comforted me. I had never felt a peace like this before, nor comfort in a long time. Growing up, I thought God was probably real, but now I was sure. I also discovered God could bring change where I or others could not. This was significant. For the first time, I felt a solid sense of hope in my soul, the kind of hope I desperately needed. Still in awe and with a quiet sense of relief, I returned to the adult psych unit the following day, changed.

Even Nurse Jaine could see the difference upon my return. She quipped in her English accent, "The Cassie I met at the start of the year wasn't very nice, but this Cassie I like." Although it wasn't the best thing she could have said, it affirmed that a profound and positive change had occurred within me. God knew exactly what factors contributed to anorexia and how depression was not only a significant factor but that underneath it, I lacked peace and hope. He alone supplied precisely what my soul had been longing for all along. Later that night, I knelt on my bed in the adult psych unit and confessed to God:

"I feel so scared at how anorexia has entered my mind and heart and taken me to dark places. I am sorry for shutting you out for so long. I need you. I need you to reign in my life."

5. Awakening

Just as hope was breaking through, Nurse Andy entered the scene. Andy consistently treated people on the eating disorder program with dignity and respect. He was firm yet flexible with the rules and let us sit away from the facility, on the grassy sports field, for afternoon tea. His approach felt affirming, helping to bring back a part of myself. I had a wonderful dietitian who was knowledgeable on anorexia, approachable and equally kind. She, too, started taking me outdoors and into the fresh air and sunshine for our appointments, gently exposing me to life beyond the disorder. I could now also join the art group, even though I hadn't gained the required weight to do so. Nervously, I created a collage of my childhood. Upon finishing, Nurse Jaine sat beside me to discuss it. Detached from self for so long through anorexia, reflecting on my up-bringing felt dreamlike. It was as though I was looking at someone else's memories—but I knew they were mine. As I meditated on each photo, my soul began to stir, and I identified with parts of my life long forgotten.

Glimpse of Freedom

Inwardly, restoration was occurring, but as I was still severely under-weight, the team agreed to take a strict approach to my treatment. Nurse

Jaine sternly but caringly said, "From tomorrow, you'll need to lie still on your bed for two hours after each meal. If you can't, we'll have to sedate you. And regardless of whether you complete your meals, we're going to give you supplements through your PEG tube and drinking them is not an option." I endured unfair treatment with nurses sedating me if I moved my leg just an inch and enforcing that I stay on my bed longer than two hours. It also made no sense why I couldn't drink the supplement, which left me thinking, *Is putting it through the tube meant to serve as a punishment?* However, for the first time, unkind nurses and treatment approaches I disagreed with didn't anger me. I now felt safe knowing I was under God's care and that he was helping me. Actually, God had always been reaching out and caring for me during anorexia—through people's kind gestures and encouraging words, by keeping me safe and even in the moments when I soaked in the sunshine. I just didn't see it at the time. Yet now that I looked to him, I could see it. Sensing that I was safe in his care, freedom appeared. It wasn't instant freedom from anorexia. Instead, I felt free from distress and anxiety about treatment. Despite my circumstances, I was now able to cooperate with treatment and felt at peace that most nurses meant well. I even began looking to God when feeling compelled to engage in eating disorder behaviours, such as watering down the milk on my cereal when no one was watching. His presence felt stronger than anorexia, helping me to feel less out of control and more able to challenge the disorder. At last, the fight against eating disorder programs and staff had ended, and *the battle to overcome anorexia had begun.*

I kept taking small steps forward, so on the 23rd of December, they discharged me. I had been in three treatment facilities straight, along with brief stays in medical wards, totalling over a year of inpatient treatment with scarcely any leave. I was then stepped down, not to a day program, but straight home.

As the new year began, I gathered my schoolbooks and packed a lunch I hoped didn't look too odd for my first day at my new senior high. I felt disappointed that I missed out on graduating and celebrating the end of schooling with my friends, who all finished school the previous year. Yet, I was grateful to attend a senior high that catered to mature-aged students and offered a flexible part-time approach to schooling.

Returning to school felt both good and strange. Being around other young people felt refreshing, even though it seemed like we were worlds apart. I enjoyed the mental stimulation that learning provided despite my capacity to concentrate being next to zero. I even liked it when the boys misbehaved and were cheeky during class. Before anorexia, I didn't take notice of boys mucking up, but now I appreciated a bit of fun, a spark of joy. Being treated with respect and like a "normal" person also felt deeply affirming after being treated and feeling like "just an anorexic" for so long.

Life outside also meant eating without nurses overseeing mealtimes, which felt surreal after being under constant watch in treatment. Yet, knowing that God was with me enabled me to eat three (small) meals and snacks each day. It felt familiar to be watched and to have my eating accounted for. Sensing God's presence, rather than just the overwhelming pull of anorexia, controlling what I could and couldn't eat, think, feel or do, also allowed me to feel safe when attempting to eat.

Weigh-ins as an outpatient further gave me a reason to keep up my intake with the threat of hospitalisation if my weight dropped. Unlike some people with anorexia, I never intended to lose more weight, so at least this wasn't an area of conflict for me. Still, I was often relieved when I did lose weight because it meant I could allow myself to eat a little more.

Over-exercising was also still an issue. I compulsively walked each day, no matter the weather or if I were sick, yet I made some progress in this area too. I could now stop walking after a set amount of time without too much of a struggle. However, I still couldn't break free from having to stand almost all the time during waking hours. I only allowed myself to sit down if I had to, like in a classroom, travelling in a car or at dinnertime. At my worst, I couldn't even do that. One time, Mum picked me up from the unit to visit Ma, who had suffered a stroke. I hysterically cried as she drove to the nursing home and wouldn't stop moving my legs. So, I had made some progress, though, to outsiders, it may have seemed otherwise.

As it turns out, recovery has many layers. Standing at the school gate one afternoon, I felt the warmth of the sunshine on my back and momentarily relaxed. The next instant, I felt scared that I had allowed myself to be at ease and enjoy something. It may seem strange that enjoying the sunshine now felt difficult, whereas I savoured any chance to feel it during hospital stays. But the more I came alive within and connected with life around me, the more every step forward felt real and challenging on a whole different level.

Between Life and Death

Over the coming weeks, still having a long way to travel towards health and complete freedom, I lost weight. Yet, this time was different. I sought help and voluntarily admitted myself to a private hospital. I had to wear a heart monitor as tests showed elevated cardiac results, and my blood pressure was very low. Once my heart got the all-clear, they transferred me to the adult psych unit.

At the adult psych unit, my "second home," my body started to breakdown. My muscles became wasted again. I fell flat onto my back when pulling the covers back on my bed and couldn't get up without help. At night I became incontinent, and in the mornings I nearly blacked out with low blood sugar levels. My ankles swelled, purple spots broke out on my stomach, and I developed a sore throat. I also started having difficulty breathing. I told my doctor on more than one occasion about my breathing but felt unheard. Eventually, they sent me for an x-ray and found I had pneumonia.

While all this was happening, Mum re-admitted herself to the private psych hospital with anorexia and anxiety. At the same time, Dad was experiencing marital problems and growing depression. So, he wasn't up to talking, and I couldn't speak to Mum whenever needed.

Soon after, Dad and my stepmother divorced, and she and my sister moved interstate. It didn't affect me at the time because anorexia was still consuming most of my life. On reflection, however, I wish I had been available for my sister to talk with and spend time together during her teens. Gradually, the disorder had stolen everything good in my life. And it continued to try, but I was re-gaining ground and wasn't about to give up. Little did I know, however, that I would soon be fighting for my life.

I started having coughing attacks and couldn't complete my meals. I now readily accepted supplement drinks, which was a first. I knew I was extremely sick. I feared the state my body was in and did all I could, within the limits of the disorder, to eat, rest and stay positive.

One night, struggling to breathe, I tried to call out for a nurse. I felt scared. Another patient heard me and asked a nurse to help, only to have her say, "Don't listen to Cassie. She is only doing it for attention." I had been a patient there for a long time and had never called out, so it should have made them think something was wrong. Yet, with the common misconception that people with anorexia are attention-seeking, my cry for help went unheard. My stepdad visited that week, and even he could easily see how sick I was. He phoned the unit after he left to speak to a nurse, expressing his concern for my health. In the years to come, his eyes would well up with tears when he recalled that visit.

The same week, I told a nurse on the eating disorder team that I had chest pain. To my relief, she believed me and responded straight away. I had an electrocardiogram (ECG), and the doctor ordered another chest x-ray and bronchoscopy. The bronchoscopy required that I fast before the procedure. I felt faint, yet as I watched the nurse about to hang up a bag of IV fluids, I asked, "Do I have to have the fluids?" I thought it might have dextrose, a form of sugar that equated in my mind to calories. I wanted the fluids. I knew how sick I was, but anorexia still had a firm grip on me, and I felt compelled to question her, hoping she would enforce it. She didn't. I went in for the procedure without the IV fluids. They then sedated me, but I was aware when they began guiding the scope down my throat. Drowsy, I managed a few swear words to communicate I wasn't asleep. It was painful and scary. They upped the anaesthesia dose and the procedure went ahead.

On returning to the unit, a doctor explained that I needed an NG tube as I was becoming weaker and unable to complete meals. He even allowed me to insert the tube myself, as it was less painful that way. I must admit, for the first time, I felt grateful to have one.

After dinner, I asked my nurse, "Could you help me stand up?" He just laughed, saying, "I'm sure you can do it yourself," and walked away. Too weak to stand up, I sat at the dining table for a long hour until a patient helped me.

Thankfully, a trainee nurse could see how sick I was and did something about it. Edward kindly set up a chair for me with blankets and pillows in the bathroom and ran a hot shower to create steam to help ease my breathing. It meant a lot to be seen and cared for.

I stood outside the nurses' station each night that week until I was about to fall asleep. I felt scared being alone in my room. If I had difficulty breathing or stopped breathing altogether, no one would know. One night, I was coughing up blood and not just tiny streaks. Frightened, I knocked on the nurses' station door, only to have them say, "Go away." With utter exhaustion and desperation, I resorted to phoning Mum on the patient's phone and told her I was coughing up blood and asked if she could call the nurses to inform them.

Mum called the nurses' station, and a nurse responded, "I'm sure it wouldn't be blood."

"Have you checked?"

"I'm sure it wouldn't be blood," she repeated.

They never did check.

Between standing at the nurses' station at night and sitting up in bed trying to breathe, I had two vivid dreams. One was of hell. Hell was a place separate from life. It was pitch black with a red haze, and the atmosphere felt heavy and thick. As my eyes adjusted to the darkness, I saw the spirits of people passing by. I wanted to talk to them, but I had a deep all-knowing that they didn't speak because words were pointless now. I saw and felt a place beyond sadness; it was of utter, endless hopelessness. I wanted to get out of there but knew once I was there, it was too late. My other dream was of heaven. The part of heaven I found myself in looked like a lush green tropical rainforest. The flowers differed from those on Earth; they looked and felt more alive, and even the waterfall gushed with living water. The only person I saw there was my stepdad. Again, no words were spoken, but for the opposite reason, there was such contentment, peace, a sense of wellbeing and a knowing on a deeper level. Here, I could have stayed.

I wondered why I had these dreams, *Perhaps my fear of dying triggered the dream of hell? While peace in knowing my destiny gave me a glimpse into heaven?* I was unsure.

What I know, however, is that following these dreams, I found myself in a very real near-death experience. On the 19th of March, the siren on the oxygen saturation monitor attached to my finger rang. My nurse responded by mumbling, "Stupid machine," and unplugged it from the wall. Soon after, another nurse came by and re-checked my oxygen levels, which were reading a dangerously low 60% (oxygen sats need to be 95-100% anything less warrants immediate medical intervention). The nurse decided the readings were correct and arranged my transfer to the hospital. I was relieved to receive help, yet anxious about the change in my plans and routine. Eventually, a couple of wardsmen arrived and escorted me on a stretcher in the dark of the night by the underground route of the hospital to the emergency department. Laying on the hard stretcher, watching the fluorescent hospital lights flash overhead, I concentrated on breathing in and out—in and out. I felt moments away from dying.

Once in the emergency department, I told myself, I had much to look forward to. *I haven't been kissed, swum with dolphins or been in a hot-air balloon yet.* I did all I could to stay positive and alive. They didn't give me a buzzer, so I called out for help when I couldn't breathe, to which I heard a nurse say to another, "Don't worry, she just wants attention." Like many people with anorexia, attention was the last thing I usually wanted, but now I wanted attention—medical attention.

The morning came, and the nurse found me in a mess. I had brown sputum down the front of me and was incontinent. She scorned, "Look, you've made a disgrace of yourself." I was too sick to care about her comment. I was more concerned about my sugar levels not being checked and not having any IV fluids or my heart monitored. No one called my parents through the night to inform them of my critical state. It was merely because it was Mum's birthday that she came to visit, only to find me in the emergency department. Her birthday just became one of the worst days of her life.

Nurse Jaine visited. "Here, Cassie, have a drink. You absolutely need it." I hadn't been offered any food or drink until now, though I felt nearly unconscious. My doctor from the adult psych unit also visited. She held my hand, saying, "Sorry, I didn't know how sick you were." Although I showed many clear signs of being severely ill, I didn't once spike a fever, which confused matters as to how to treat me. Later, an international health journal documented that in rare cases, like mine, people with severe anorexia react differently to bacterial infections because their immune systems are already so compromised. The head psychiatrist returned from leave and gently explained, "We'll get you moved upstairs, where they'll take care of you."

After two blood transfusions, staff lifted me from the emergency department bed to another bed. They didn't support my head when lifting, and it flung back. I think they didn't realise how weak I was. My neck hurt, and I cried in pain. Before reaching the ward, they transferred me onto another bed to have an MRI (magnetic resonance imaging) of my chest, and again, I cried in pain (years later, an osteopath diagnosed me with a neck injury, likely sustained by the unsupported transfer). The MRI revealed upper and lower lobe bacterial pneumonia in my right lung, with thick mucus and an abscess in the middle lobe. Ordinarily, they would operate and drain the abscess, but I was too underweight for that, with my weight dropping to the lowest it had ever been. I looked severely emaciated and felt incredibly sick. Mum was warned, with the words no parent wants to hear: "Be prepared for her not to make it."

Late that night, the doctor on duty inserted a central line into my neck for the direct and aggressive administration of antibiotics. He was warm and kind, like a concerned father. People like him stood out to me.

The next day, medical staff planned to rapidly refeed me so I could gain weight for the operation to go ahead. The eating disorder team, however, halted their plan. I overheard my dietitian telling the staff that rapid refeeding could trigger a heart attack and I wouldn't survive. Their only solution was to keep going with the IV antibiotics and hope for the best.

The medical staff also put up a bag of IV dextrose, yet when the eating disorder team learnt of this, they quickly stopped the dextrose and replaced it with sodium chloride. The dextrose could have also provoked refeeding complications.

I felt hard-pressed on every side. Morning and night, I swallowed over twenty pills and had just as many tubes of blood collected. I had oedema and minimal muscle power in my neck and legs. Pressure sores broke out on my back. I was also incontinent with diarrhoea. Two elderly patients that I shared the room with weren't understanding. In disgust, one told me, whilst the other agreed, "You should clean the bathroom after every use." I could hardly breathe or walk, let alone clean a bathroom.

Seeing the physiotherapist each day was both a relief and an anxiety-filled event, full of dread and fear. The physio was gentle and kind and openly shared how she had recovered from anorexia herself. Yet, I had to lay down for the exercises, which made it extremely difficult to breathe and left me feeling thoroughly exhausted and in pain all over.

Mum and Dad took turns visiting and sitting with me for meal support. I even let Mum massage my feet and asked Dad to lay my pillows in a specific position each night to help me breathe more easily. Other people visited too, but unintentionally, they only added to my exhaustion. I felt out of breath and drained with making eye contact and small talk. On the other hand, receiving cards and flowers was a sweet blessing I now welcomed.

Then, just when we thought it couldn't get any worse, it did. I contracted blood poisoning *candida septicaemia* through the central line. I was now spiking fevers and felt unbearably cold. They feared this alone could kill me. The doctor quickly removed the central line and after multiple painful attempts, inserted a long line in my arm. My zinc and potassium levels were low, so I had a drip for these too. Being this sick was incredibly scary. Night-time was the worst. I sat up every night and stayed awake as long as I could, fearing that if I fell asleep, I would stop breathing, which was a real possibility.

The likelihood of me surviving this admission was not in my favour. My parents still believed in God, and Mum knew I needed a miracle. She phoned family and friends, asking them to pray for me. Years later, I discovered a prayer Mum had written. It reads:

"God, I pray for you to heal my daughter of pneumonia and heal her psychologically and physically of anorexia. I ask you to give me the strength to keep going and for people to support me. I ask for faith to believe you can do all things. I am praying for a miracle."

God doesn't always answer prayers the way we expect him to, but he answered with a direct miracle this time. I gained a little weight, my electrolytes re-balanced and my fever subsided. Although physically weak, I was strong inside and didn't lose faith. I kept encouraging myself to eat and rest. I prayed often, and Mum wheelchaired me to the hospital chapel on Sundays.

Against all odds, pneumonia cleared, and they transferred me back to the adult psych unit. The respiratory team came to the unit to follow up on my progress. When they saw me, they were surprised. The doctor said, "It is remarkable you are alive and doing so well."

My weight also improved without the help of an NG tube, so the team decided I could step down to a day program. Nurse Jaine, with a smile, said I would now live in an apartment block around the corner from a day program with another young woman, Dana, who also had anorexia.

Living with Dana allowed different aspects of life to break through. I enjoyed re-arranging our lounge room, making it homely by placing a cane basket full of books, candles and coloured wool on our coffee table. Dana and I had fun wagging the day program at times, watching *Neighbours* on the telly, sharing a meal (in a fashion) and staying up late talking. It was good to have more freedom and to feel like a young adult. Dana also invited a few girls from the program over to hang out, drink, smoke pot and swap pills. To my benefit, the mere thought of calories in alcohol and feeling a loss of self-control with drugs kept me in my room, politely declining to join in. Besides, I was starting to feel alive within and didn't need drugs anyway.

With life seeping through and spending weekends at home, I looked forward to celebrating my nineteenth birthday with Tanya. Mum shouted us a Harley-Davidson joy ride through the mountains, and we wrapped up the day by playing carnival games at our local annual fair. It certainly was an improvement on my last birthday! The day after, the family of a friend of mine from the adolescent psych unit dropped by (my friend was now in prison, but we kept in contact through letters). They had a gift for me, a painting of two dolphins finding their way through the depths of the sea. No longer fearing gifts, I warmly accepted the artwork my friend's father had created and eagerly hung the canvas on my bedroom wall.

Spending weekends at home also meant I could attend church. At church one morning, I sensed I should pray with someone for Dana. It went against where I was at. It meant being me for that moment and not bound by anorexia. I walked out of the church, but the inner prompting was so strong that I turned around, walked back in and found the youth leader to pray with. Returning to our apartment the next day, I learnt that around the time we prayed for Dana her life was in danger. Dana had collapsed, and without knowing this, a mutual friend suddenly felt she should drop by and check on her. Finding Dana in a compromised state, our friend sought medical attention and potentially saved her life. Later, when Dana returned from the hospital, I told her I had prayed for her and believed God had intervened through our friend to keep her safe. In her Irish accent, she confessed, "You know, Cas, I was uncertain about us living together, but you've turned out to be the best flatmate I could have had."

Searching Deeper

Apart from time spent with Dana, participating in cognitive behavioural therapy (CBT) and guided visualisation groups, my memory of the day program is hazy. I do recall, however, the clinical director asking,

"What would you be doing if you didn't have anorexia?"

"I think I'd be doing mission work, helping the poor," came my reply.

It was a simple question, yet no one had asked it before. It was also a powerful question. Something deep within my heart stirred, and I felt seen and affirmed.

The next day, I asked the director, "Have you seen the movie *Labyrinth?*"

He kind of nodded.

"Well, there's a girl. She's in a maze and on a mission to find and save her baby brother. In one scene, she finds herself in her childhood bedroom, with all her pretty ornaments, precious photos and cherished belongings. Yet, it isn't really her bedroom. It's just an illusion, an enticement to make her forget the real mission." I'm not sure he knew where I was going with it all until I added, "I think the world is like that."

"In what way?" he asked.

"It tries to distract you from what truly matters and keeps you from seeing what's really going on. Society keeps you busy, materialism makes you feel good and the media dictates how we see things. I don't want to be a part of that."

He listened, then said, "I think anorexia is like that. Anorexia is like the girl's bedroom with all the illusions and distractions keeping you from the real world."

True. Yet it wasn't what I was getting at. Anorexia had helped me separate from the world. It had gotten me out of things I felt locked into, gave me time to ponder what truly counts and allowed me to no longer care about fitting in. I didn't want to let it go, only to return to a world I had escaped from. Instead, I wanted to continue on the spiritual path, which offered a new outlook and way of life, but I didn't know how to outside of the disorder. But that's what I was after—the path of life, not an illusion.

Positive Change

Before long, the summer holidays arrived, so day program treatment ended. I saw the clinical director as an outpatient, along with a local doctor who had an interest and some training in eating disorders. I felt grateful to have good outpatient support. My doctor liaised with the eating disorder team and monitored my blood pressure, chemistry levels and weight. Just as importantly, he treated me with dignity and respect. He asked how I was feeling, chattered about everyday life and addressed any health concerns I raised—helping me to feel cared for, safe and supported.

As 2001 began, I focused on completing my final year of schooling. Being underweight made it difficult to concentrate during class, and I slept through countless lessons. I also recalled little from schooling past ninth grade, and suddenly, I had to be up to the Higher School Certificate performance level. Both my principal and teachers were aware of my position and offered support. My music teacher and a friend even came to my home and provided free piano lessons, helping me to complete the work and pass the exams.

Inwardly, I also kept making progress, yet anorexia was still strong, and brief admissions to the adult psych unit during the school term were frequent. In all honesty, I now found it a relief to be admitted when my energy levels and eating were dropping at home. Treatment helped me to rest and eat a bit more when I couldn't on my own. I took schoolwork to the unit, and a hospital teacher came by now and then to help with the lessons. The eating disorder team were also more flexible with my treatment now, giving me regular leave and not forcing weight gain. *Had they given up on me? Or were they trying a new approach?* I wondered. Either way, it allowed me to keep finding and connecting with life and kept me from losing more weight in the process. I could also attend chapel services, which gave me something to look forward to. I remember Nurse Evie phoning the unit on her weekend off to ensure staff were aware to allow me to go to chapel. Evie was the new head nurse on the eating disorder program and was warm-hearted and understanding. She told me, "I love nursing," and it showed. With proper training in eating disorders coupled with her compassion, consistency and firmness, she made me feel supported and cared for.

The program had also improved, with music, cooking and dietetic groups now available. They even allowed me to bring a CD player into my room, and I began listening and dancing to worship music. I still didn't feel happy and couldn't let myself laugh or be silly, but I now felt an inner joy when playing the music. I also made friends with a couple of eating disorder patients who were Christians and taking steps forward, making for a positive atmosphere. I remained underweight and struggled to eat all my food and rest, so it wasn't easy, but because of my rekindled faith and the changes made to treatment, these admissions felt somewhat helpful now.

Between admissions, there was still much adjusting to do. I watched people while waiting for a bus, wondering, *How do they get up each day, eat, go shopping, catch a bus home, and do it all over again the next day?* I also walked by a sports field, saw people with picnic rugs and water bottles, and gazed upon the colours and textures, thinking, *I haven't seen these for so long. They look so colourful and shiny.* I had forgotten such things existed.

Being in public places, however, like the local mall, was challenging. I had to tell myself, *Put one foot in front of the other and keep walking.* I shook when speaking to people or just walking by them. I had become so institutionalised and detached from society and self that re-integrating proved to be a more involved process than anticipated. Hearing my friends talk about movies, worldwide news events and the latest music also felt strange. I hadn't watched television or listened to the radio for several years and still didn't, so I had no idea what they were talking about. Even years later, when people referred to a big news event that occurred during my eating disorder, it was like I was in a time warp, and it never happened.

As the year went on, our high school graduation day arrived. At twenty years old, I finally completed my schooling. Mum and Dad came to the graduation, and we had our photo taken together, the first picture of all three of us since they divorced. It felt healing having both my parents there together.

It wasn't long, however, until I was reminded that all was not well. Standing in line to receive my graduation certificate, a student I didn't know asked, "Are you okay?" Then proceeded to say, "You look too thin." It didn't bother me. I understood her concern. I was used to people I didn't know stopping me in the street or shopping centres and telling me I needed to get better. A man approached me in the supermarket one time and said in an urgent but gentle manner, "My wife died from anorexia. I know it's hard to recover, but you need to." I knew these people were right, so after graduation, it was back to the adult psych unit for me.

During this "recoup" admission, I made friends with a middle-aged man with anorexia. With his gentle and caring nature, he painted a picture of teddy bears gazing at flowers during art therapy for me. He also believed in God, so one time, we even prayed for another patient while standing in the corridor. Throughout treatment, I also met younger men, as well as older women with the disorder, and people from all different backgrounds and cultures. It wasn't just young white women receiving treatment for anorexia, as often portrayed in the media.

I also enjoyed getting to know the general psych patients as well. I made friends with Leo, a man who thought I was Alanis Morissette. He critiqued performances he believed I gave, and in return, I smiled, nodded and went along with it all. I read daily devotions to an elderly man, Johnston, and ensured he didn't miss out on his tea and toast. I made friends with Teresa, whose home was now on the streets despite being Australia's first female surgeon many years ago. I often talked with another lady, Rosie, over a black coffee. Rosie struggled with depression and was receiving electric shock therapy. Sam/Samantha, who crossdressed, gave me a pink floral lipstick case out of the kindness of his heart. I made friends with Jack, a man in a wheelchair who was delusional. He called me his Scottish angel.

Jack would say, "Hey Cas, can you get me a 2SM?" Which I learnt meant a coffee with two sugars and milk.

To which I'd reply, "Get your own 2SM Jack." We joked around. It was good.

There were still moments, however, when I felt unsafe residing with other patients. For instance, a lady decided she was me and believed I was an impersonator. She didn't like that and told me off. A patient also came into my room while I was asleep. She crouched in the corner and tried to light a cigarette. I woke because of a rustling noise.

In the dark, I cautiously asked, "Who's there?"

An unfamiliar voice whispered, "I can't go outside to smoke, and I can't smoke in my room. I just want to smoke."

"You can't smoke in my room either. There are smoke detectors."

"I won't be long."

"No, you need to leave. You're scaring me."

After repeating, "Please leave," a couple more times, she did. It was pretty crazy, but because I was feeling more centred, other patients' mental states and behaviours no longer overwhelmed me. I liked these people. They were intelligent, caring, interesting and easy to talk with.

Back home, my friends started getting ready for our twelfth grade formal (or prom, as some call it). I had missed out on the tenth and twelfth grade formals at my previous school, so now I could make up for it. My doctor at the unit, however, didn't want me to go. I knew I was very underweight but reasoned that *Surely one night at the formal would be more beneficial than another night in the psych unit.* The doctor let me voice my opinion but made it clear that with my low weight, he didn't approve of me going and thought it a ridiculous thing to do. Nevertheless, he let me go.

Once home, I bought a black and gold halter neck dress that needed taking in. I knew how thin I looked, so I bought a large tin of protein powder. I stirred water into it and secretly ate the mixture over the next two nights, which was dangerous. With a sudden and high intake of calories, my electrolyte levels could have shifted, and I could have gone into cardiac failure and died from refeeding syndrome.[6] Although I was aware of this and knew a lady who was rumoured to have died from refeeding, I did it anyway. I was desperate and starving. Thankfully, I didn't go into cardiac failure. Still, my body couldn't cope with the overload of calories, and I ended up dehydrated and looking and feeling worse for it. It would have been far better if I had eaten normally and rested the two days beforehand, but I couldn't let myself. None of this stopped me from going to the formal though. I was determined to go.

Fiona, who I had been friends with since seventh grade, braided my hair. Dad pinned a crystal rose pendant onto my dress. My parents took photos and made me feel loved and supported. I went to the formal too unwell and exhausted to enjoy it. I neither felt nor looked attractive, being severely underweight. I also found it anxiety-provoking to eat with my peers. Yet, I was glad I went and finished my schooling with everyone else.

On return to the psych unit, I talked with my nurse about the formal. She confessed, "I never went to mine. I didn't think I was pretty enough." I could see the sadness in her eyes, and it impacted me. *She was pretty. How could she not see that? And it shouldn't have mattered anyway what she looked like.* I also knew how she felt. In the past, I had wanted to hide because of my appearance, but now I didn't feel quite the same. Something within was changing.

6. Dawn

Life was looking a little brighter as 2002 began, and like any high school graduate, I started contemplating my career path and which courses to take. I still had an interest in helping people in developing countries. So, I enrolled in a diploma of intercultural studies through distance education with Tabor College. I felt more optimistic about my future. But, struggling with anorexia, I continued receiving support at the adult psych unit this year too.

One admission, a professor specialising in eating disorders visiting from the UK remarked, "You are the most stuck patient I have ever seen." Although I was making inward progress, I wasn't going forward or backward weight-wise. My doctor at the unit also thought I was "stuck" and wanted me to take anti-anxiety medication to help with OCD. I declined the medication, but he kept encouraging me to take it, so I agreed. I didn't want to be difficult again. Yet I never swallowed the pills, I only pretended to. Although I knew medication helped others, I was scared it would make me relax and gain weight without working through the thoughts and emotions behind anorexia. I also feared returning to my natural weight and losing the "self-discipline" I had developed.

Alternative Path

Coincidently, while in the adult psych unit, I had to read the book *Celebration of Discipline* by Richard J. Foster[7] for intercultural studies. As I read, I reflected how before anorexia, I felt out of control and ruled and pulled by my appetite, emotions and desires, much of which I deemed "bad." I longed to feel clean, free and at peace. I identified with people who engaged with Buddhism, orthorexia[8] and who ventured into the wilderness to leave society and themselves behind. However, meditating on Foster's teachings, I saw my longings were valid but that self-discipline based on self-criticism and deception only suppressed my appetite, emotions and desires. My own effort at self-discipline also didn't bring me closer to God or unlock true purity, freedom or peace. In fact, it was a false sense of spirituality I was engaging in because God was not a part of it. With further reading, I found the Bible explains how self-control, similar to self-discipline, is a fruit of the spirit (Galatians 5:22-23). This made me think: *Fruit does not appear overnight. Fruit takes time to grow, and like a tree, I only need to put down deep roots in God's love and truth, and like a gardener, he prunes, waters and looks after the tree.*

My own attempt at self-discipline was harsh, propelled by lies and brought detachment not only from self but from other people, God, and therefore life itself. It also hindered self-control from flourishing and allowed fear to rule. By contrast, I was seeing that healthy self-discipline is the beautiful by-product of an intimate relationship with our maker and serves to release life, not take it. With this insight came further hope—hope that there is an alternative to self-discipline via starvation and rules and that the alternative is better, in every way.

Not long after, a friend quoted me a scripture passage. The passage is about a rich man who asks, "What must I do to inherit eternal life?" Jesus tells him to keep the commandments. The man says he has. Jesus loves this man. He tells him to sell his possessions and give the money to the poor, and then he will have treasure in heaven, and when he has done this, to come and follow him. The rich man finds this hard to do and walks away. Jesus' disciples then question him about this incident (Mark 10:17-26).

When I heard this passage, I thought I was like the rich man, and I had to let go of anorexia to be a Christian, which deeply troubled me. I needed God's help in the first place to let go of anorexia—I couldn't do it on my own. I wasn't even sure if I wanted to recover anyhow. Left with a heavy heart and a racing mind, I wondered: *Am I displeasing to God? Am I even a Christian? Does this mean I am resigned to living separately from God for eternity?*

It wasn't until sometime later that I read the entire chapter and found it says, "Then who in the world can be saved?" they asked. Jesus looked at them intently and said, "Humanly speaking, it is impossible. But not with God. Everything is possible with God" (Mark 10:27 New Living Translation, NLT).

Growing up, I learnt the basics about God and my relationship with him. So, I understood God is the Father, Son and Spirit. I also knew that humanity once lived in a perfect world, with our perfect God. And yet, all this changed when we chose to know both good and evil, despite God's warning. As a result, our relationship with our creator became broken, and death and darkness entered the world. I further understood that God loved the world—so Jesus, the Son, came to earth to restore all that was broken by living in perfect union with the Father and freely sacrificing his life on the cross, on behalf of humankind, for all our wrongdoings. Then, by rising from the dead, he showed that even death and darkness no longer had power over humanity. I also knew that if I trusted Jesus and relied on what he has done for us, I could know God and eternal life.

Yet, although I knew all of this, I didn't understand its implications. Being underweight didn't help with seeing things clearly either. So, you can imagine the relief I felt when I grasped the truth that *regardless of my brokenness and sin, I can have a relationship with God and know life to the fullest—because he alone has made it possible.*

The more I tasted truths, the more I sought and found them. A few days later, while trying to allow myself to increase my intake, all I heard and felt was torment, so I asked God to show me things as they really are. Later that same day, while on leave for a few hours from the unit, a shopkeeper said, "You're all bones. You need to eat more and be well." Through finding truths that spoke to my soul, the path before me continued to light up, revealing not my deepest fears but the way to life.

Seeing and Caring

Still in the adult psych unit, I had a special visit from my big sister. She was in town for business, yet hurried from the train station to see me. Living interstate, we had seen little of each other over the years, but my sister wrote letters and posted photos of herself and her girls, helping us to stay connected. So, I felt heartened upon her arrival, yet also embarrassed. *I look so underweight, and I'm in a psych unit,* I thought to myself. However, it didn't bother my sister. She sat on my bed, hugged me, accepted me as I was and we chatted. Although the visit was short, it felt good to see her and to know I had a big sister I could be myself with and who loved me unconditionally.

Sadly, however, not all people in the psych unit had caring support. I distinctly recall one man pacing the corridor and circling the lone tree in the courtyard for days, from morning to night (someone with anorexia notices these things). A lightning storm struck when he was still pacing around the tree. I knew his name, so I looked on the allocation board to see who his nurse was and went and told her,

"Joe's outside pacing in the storm."

"Don't worry about him," she replied.

I felt distressed seeing him being left outside, all alone, in the fierce storm. Yet, I didn't feel angry at the nurse. I knew she was busy, and I felt comforted, even empowered, knowing I could ask God for help. So, from inside the unit, looking out, I prayed. I asked God to calm Joe's soul and said aloud, "Whatever is causing him to walk nonstop must leave."

Just as I finished praying, he walked inside the unit and sat down. God sees and cares.

My family and friends see and care too. I was discharged a few days before my twenty-first birthday, and with an unusual sense of excitement, I organised a fancy-dress party. We hired a hall, catering and a jukebox and decked the place with pink and orange balloons.

People from all areas of my life rocked up. Tanya and Dianna came, of course. Amber, my childhood friend from church, came too. Fiona and a bunch of other high school friends, along with Madeleine, who I hadn't seen since primary school, also made it. To my surprise, Gran, Pop and Uncle Trevor also turned up. Dad came dressed as Captain Cook, my step-dad a pirate and Mum a hippie. Even a couple of guys from the adolescent psych unit and a man from the adult psych unit joined the celebration. I felt incredibly blessed.

I was still struggling with anorexia, monitoring everything I ate, and I didn't eat any of my birthday cake, but my world was changing. I now loved being around people and organising parties, like I used to. Even though I had pushed family and friends away through the disorder or disengaged from doing life with them, they saw beyond and kept loving me regardless.

Wise Mind

As the year progressed, still classified as having severe anorexia and needing ongoing support, I returned to the adult psych unit. I hadn't had individual therapy at this facility, even though I had been a patient there on and off for four years, but that was about to change. They offered me to see a clinician specifically trained in eating disorders, and I accepted the offer. To my relief, this clinician was caring, easy to talk with and understood eating disorders. I liked meeting with her. She took an interest in the course I was studying by distance education and explored how I could regain living skills such as shopping and cooking to prepare for returning home. One session, she asked, "Why don't you consider trying a day program again?" I knew day programs expected normal eating, weight restoration and complete recovery. However, I was still content to recover in small steps and to the limit I allowed myself. Complete recovery was not on my soon-to-do list. I felt overwhelmed and scared by the mere thought of letting go of my highly ordered world. Anorexia felt familiar, and besides, returning to my natural weight was unappealing. I didn't like how I looked or felt before my eating disorder, so why would I want to return to that? Even though I didn't want to have anorexia forever, I couldn't imagine life without it.

The clinician counselling me then took leave, and I saw another lady, a psychologist. With her sincerity, compassion and sound insight into anorexia, she also made me feel safe and supported. She took the approach of getting me to ask, "What does my wise mind say?" As simple and perhaps as silly as it sounds, it proved helpful. "Wise mind" considered "reason mind" and "emotional mind" thoughts but allowed wisdom to form conclusions on matters. For example, if I was tossing up whether to eat the dessert (which was on my meal plan), rather than giving a calculated "reason mind" response such as, "I am gaining enough weight without eating dessert, so why should I eat it?" Listening to my heart or "wise mind" let me say, "I think eating dessert now and then is fine; no matter my weight, it's good to have a treat." It didn't mean my "wise" answers always resulted in action, but sometimes they did. As a result, my black-and-white, fear dominated thinking that had become so ingrained took a backseat. I also found the process itself, which was a part of dialectical behaviour therapy (DBT), of engaging with wisdom rather than tackling eating disordered thoughts with logic and reason, was refreshing and helped me gain a further sense of self.

I am unsure how it happened, but after seeing this new psychologist, I found myself leaving the adult psych unit to start the day program.

The 17th of January 2003 was my first day at this day program. Unlike other treatment programs, it was run inside an old brick house surrounded by green lawns and tall oak trees, offering a healthful environment away from the hospital grounds. Weighing less than I did when I first entered treatment six years ago, I was kindly but firmly told, "You're too underweight to be here, but we'll have you on the program if you follow the guidelines and meet the eating and weight gain requirements. If you can't do this, we'll admit you straight to hospital." The clinical director also informed me I needed to stop my college degree and put all my focus on recovery. I wasn't keen on any of this. I felt angry that they wanted me to defer my studies, the one "normal" aspect of my life. Yet, they seemed supportive and wanted the best for me, so I gave their program a go.

The program ran Monday to Friday, from morning tea to dinnertime. Mum drove me to the station, where I caught a train, then a bus and walked a short distance to the program, back and forth each day. The meals served were high quality, generous in serving size and included "challenging" foods like cakes, quiches and apple pies. I had to sit with the other patients and our nurse for each meal and snack. They expected us to eat normally; this meant using regular-sized cutlery, not dissecting food or eating painfully slow. I had to gain at least 0.5 kilograms per week until I reached a BMI of 20. They had a "three strikes and you're out" system, so if I didn't complete a meal or gain weight three times, I had to leave the program.

Groups constantly ran when it wasn't mealtime. The groups looked at various aspects of recovery, from challenging thoughts and learning to identify and sit with emotions to dietetic lessons, self-care, goal setting, body image, communication skills and more. We had one-on-one meetings with the dietitian, our therapist (I continued seeing the same psychologist from the adult psych unit) and the program director.

The day program was so full on that after the first few days, I thought of five good reasons why I should leave the program and never return. At the same time, I had been struggling with the fact that I was allowing myself to attend a program that may very well help me recover. What to do? The eating disorder part of me didn't want to stay, the part of me that didn't like aspects of the program also didn't want to stay, but something in my spirit felt I should. Unable to decide, I prayed, "God, I need your help. Can you show me if I should stay or leave the program?" The next day, one by one, my reasons for leaving the program were addressed and undone. Being left with no reasons to go and only signs to stay, I pressed on.

Recovering Body and Soul

As I stayed on, I found this program fostered a caring atmosphere with highly dedicated and well-trained staff. It wasn't perfect, but it was the best treatment I had experienced by far. We also had the same two nurses join us at mealtimes and groups daily, providing consistency in care. Nurse Tia, in particular, helped me to feel nurtured and supported. She would notice if I were down or struggling and with genuine concern would ask, "What's going on for you, Miss Cassie? How can I help?"

Feeling well-supported, I made continual efforts to push past my set limits and comfort zone with eating, weight gain and connecting to life. It wasn't easy. It meant eating more than what felt helpful, feeling so full that it was uncomfortable and sitting in groups all day without an exercise program. Attending also meant voicing my thoughts and feelings while eating and gaining weight. It was physically, mentally and emotionally exhausting. Most of all, it meant change. I knew I was slowly but surely recovering in my body and soul. I even started being kind to myself, and for my twenty-second birthday, I gave myself twenty-two self-caring gifts:

1. I allow myself to paint

2. I allow myself to do craft

3. I allow myself to play the keyboard

4. I allow myself to read novels

5. I allow myself to read magazines

6. I allow myself to read newspapers

7. I allow myself to light candles

8. I allow myself to listen to my favourite music

9. I allow myself to use my foot spa

10. I allow myself to use my comfortable pillow

11. I allow myself to ask for massages

12. I allow myself to put bag(s) down whilst travelling

13. I allow myself to play with my dogs

14. I allow myself to play computer games

15. I allow myself to paint my nails

16. I allow myself to shower at anytime

17. I allow myself to play skill testers

18. I allow myself to wear UGG boots

19. I allow myself to sit in the company of others

20. I allow myself to sit at the bus stop

21. I allow myself to nap if unwell

22. I allow myself not to exercise if sick

Along with self-care, another avenue of healing opened up. Walking by a paddock one fresh morning, I saw a horse in the distance and stopped. I rarely stopped while on my walks. I picked some grass and watched the horse enthusiastically gallop towards me. I fed, patted and talked to him. As I bonded with the horse, I felt another piece of myself return—my love for animals.

Later, I suggested to Gran, who also loved animals, that we visit *Australia's Wildlife Park*. When I was five, I went there on my first school excursion and loved it. I had also barely seen Gran since anorexia, so I thought it would be an ideal way to reconnect. We walked around the shady nature reserve, patting and feeding the kangaroos. Being underweight, I felt exhausted and kept thinking about the next meal, but for moments in time, anorexia quietened, and my soul felt alive.

Back at the day program, I met Sharon. Sharon had anorexia, and like most of the patients, looked thin, pale and reserved. She did, however, have a noteworthy funky style about her. Sharon wore hand-knitted mittens and boots with different coloured laces and had dreads at one point too. Whenever Sharon spoke, her words were insightful and wise. She had a sense of maturity, warmth and gentleness. Through groups, I learnt she was a single mum with a young boy. Sharon walked and talked with me when our therapist took us all out to the park one day instead of having a group session, and our friendship began. Sharon befriended me when a few patients at the program shut me out. I had eating disordered behaviours that annoyed and challenged them as they battled to recover, and it was clear they disliked me because of it. However, it didn't seem to bother Sharon that I wouldn't sit to chat, even though she did.

Along with Sharon's kind nature, perhaps how anorexia affected us differently helped with building a friendship that wasn't intertwined with and dominated by the disorder. For example, Sharon would buy a Chinese meal on our lunch outing with the program, while I would always select bread with turkey and no butter (if I could get away with it). So, we had different rules and fears surrounding food. She also had the goal of not sharing her plate of food with her son but eating it all herself. I didn't have the same goal. And although anorexia affected us differently, on a spiritual level, we found common ground. We discovered we were both Christians and that hope, peace, love and joy played a significant role in our journeys.

As spirituality became a part of my everyday life, I thought more about God and the life he offers. Out on a walk one weekend, I stumbled across the word "choice." I began playing with the notion that I had a choice. Instead of "having" to eat in a certain way or set goals that abided by numbers, orders and categories, I recalled the word choice and felt able to choose in the moment how I wanted to respond. I didn't know why this word was having a profound effect on me until I discovered the spiritual reality behind it. *I did have a choice because I was already free.* I was free because Jesus set humanity free from every form of darkness that entraps and robs us of life. I had always been free, but I didn't know it tangibly until now. Stepping towards recovery suddenly seemed more doable because I didn't need to step forward into the unknown but could stand in the spiritual reality that already is. Colour was breaking forth into my black-and-white world, and I liked it. It felt good, really good.

The following week, as I sat in groups at the day program, listening to other patients share their core beliefs, I picked up on spiritual themes running through them (core beliefs are underlying beliefs about ourselves that may or may not be true). One lady with a Christian background shared that her core belief was that she was evil. As I listened to her bravely share, I wondered, *How will the team help her with her faulty belief without understanding Christianity?* I saw her many years later. She still hadn't recovered. I couldn't help but think, *If she had received spiritual support alongside treatment, perhaps her life may have looked quite different by now.*

Although the day program lacked spiritual support, the clinical director did listen to and respect my spiritual beliefs. He also had empathy yet stood firm against the eating disorder. I didn't need to explain myself and my struggle with the disorder versus recovery. He understood anorexia "worked" for me to a point, even though it was highly destructive. He made it clear that our thoughts, feelings and behaviours were not stupid or trivial but made sense, and at the same time, he equipped us through CBT to generate healthy alternate thoughts. Whenever I brought up health complaints, medical attention was promptly sought. Just as importantly, he spoke to me as Cassie rather than an eating disorder. With his care and ability to think outside the box, he directed a safe, supportive and effective program, enabling me to gain a sense of self-respect and to keep engaging in treatment that supported full recovery.

I spent the rest of the year on and off at the day program. Only once did I land myself in hospital, but not for anorexia. I was at home in the afternoon when my ankles started to swell and feel like they were on fire. I was in excruciating pain and had to be wheelchaired into the emergency department. My legs rapidly turned a dark blue. My knees swelled, and then my finger joints and elbows. Having a shower felt like nails were falling on my skin. They gave me pain relief and IV antibiotics, though no one knew what was wrong with me. After blood test results returned, the antibiotics ceased, as I didn't have a bacterial infection, but some virus, likely linked to my weakened immune system. Thankfully and mysteriously, it resolved, and through the short ordeal, my weight stayed very low but stable.

Even though my weight was low, it was the best it had been for years. Nonetheless, police officers on two occasions approached me as I looked like a suspicious person. One time, they asked, "Are you on drugs? Can I check your bag?"

"No," I replied and kept walking. After all, I was on my morning walk and wouldn't stop for anyone.

The other time, three undercover officers asked to search my bag. They said people had reported seeing someone like me hanging around houses where items were stolen. I had been clothes shopping that morning, and when the shopkeeper asked if I wanted my receipt, I casually said, "Oh no, don't worry about it," and walked out, but I felt I should go back and get it, so I did. The police thought I had stolen the clothes until they saw the receipt. I learnt two important facts that day. Firstly, I still looked very unhealthy, to the point of looking suspicious. Secondly, God is always helping me, as I believe he prompted me to return and get the receipt.

Holding onto hope, along with the truths I was collecting about God—that he sees, cares and can help, together with the life skills and dietetic facts treatment had provided, I began envisioning what recovery may look like. I opened my journal at home one evening and nervously wrote what I imagined I would feel at a slightly higher weight, then at a bit more and a bit more, until I reached a BMI of 20. I listed what I could do without anorexia and how my relationships would change. I also wrote my values and spiritual beliefs and how I might live them out. In brief, I wrote:

"Through learning how to eat and exercise healthily, I might feel better about my body once I recover. Hopefully, I'd also look my age at my natural weight. Without anorexia, I could attend my college campus and help people overseas. I could freely eat out with my friends and enjoy being social. I may even get a boyfriend! Recovery would also mean facing fears and trusting God to help me every step of the way."

After much writing and contemplating, I still wasn't keen to fully recover but felt curious and challenged to keep playing with the idea.

7. Sunrise

Shortly into the new year, while taking a break from the day program, I had another revelation, which proved decisive in my journey. The revelation was this—*I'm not just in a battle against anorexia. It's deeper. I'm in a spiritual battle.* Through discernment and reflecting on teachings, I realised that a dark reality is at work, evident in various forms of devastation on earth, including anorexia. I hated that. Finally, I found a motive for saying "no" to anorexia and "yes" to recovery. Although feeling far from excited about the prospect of recovery, I could no longer accept darkness in my life. Equipped and ready to take significant steps, I returned to the day program for support to see it through.

Back at the program, we set goals each Friday afternoon for the weekend ahead. Yet, no matter how often I set the goal to undo my enmeshment with Mum's eating and exercise, I couldn't. I'm not exactly sure how it happened, but during the recovery process, I had entangled my eating and exercise with Mum's. I couldn't eat more than Mum, before Mum, nor rest while she was doing housework. Adhering to these "rules" contained my anger towards Mum for not being free of her eating disorder. I wanted her to eat and rest "normally" so I could do so with less inner conflict, but she couldn't. I was idealistic and lacking grace, but also crying out for help. It felt so difficult to be my own person, to eat and rest in a way that was good for me, especially with anger and self-hate being triggered. It's easy to imagine that this was a major source of contention for us both. I felt stuck in this area until I had another revelation—*Comparison is not of God. He has made us unique with one-of-a-kind personalities and purposes. Comparison only divides and robs us of love for one another and ourselves.* With this truth at the forefront of my mind, I focused on my eating and resting, irrespective of Mum's. It wasn't easy and took time, but it was worth it. Our relationship became a little more peaceful, and homelife less tense.

After a year of steady progress, Mum suggested we celebrate by spending Christmas in the city. Secretly, I was impressed that this was Mum's idea. She avoided the city because of anxiety, yet she wanted to do something special for us.

The city, which was full of holidaymakers, had a festive vibe. We checked out the aquarium, hopped into sticker booths, explored the sunny harbourside and laughed as Mum walked in and out the revolving doors of the big city office blocks just for silly fun. We had a good day, well, until dinner. The hotel restaurant had a limited menu and lacked options that I felt at ease with eating. So, with anxiety and indecision, tension filled the air, and the eating disorder hampered the moment. Yet, thankfully, Mum was intent on having an enjoyable time and patiently waited until I ordered my food. To complete the day, we spent the evening on the harbourside and took photos under the tall Christmas tree in all its lights and splendour. Joy was returning to Christmas, and having a fun time was no longer something to fear.

I Just Knew I Was Free

As 2005 got underway, I returned to the day program. I kept progressing, so they stepped me down to attending just three days a week. My BMI had improved and was almost 18. I hadn't been this weight for seven years. The last time I approached a BMI of 18, I felt awful. This time, however, was different. I didn't feel happy about my weight, nor did I feel nervous or fat. I was recovering holistically, which meant my thoughts and feelings about my weight had changed. Even so, after several weeks, my weight plateaued, and so they asked me to leave the program.

I had an outpatient appointment with the day program director the following week. He said, "I'll give you another chance. I can see you are making progress, even though you didn't make the weight gain."

Yet, this time, I didn't toss up whether to attend the day program. Instead, mustering up courage, I said, "I feel like anorexia has lost its grip on me. I don't need the program."

I was still underweight and had many areas to work on, but I felt at peace, and I knew I'd go forward from here. So, day program treatment ended, and I had regular outpatient support. I saw the same psychologist I had been seeing for almost two years, a dietitian and my local doctor.

To celebrate, I got a dove tattooed on my shoulder blade. The dove is flying free and represents peace and new beginnings. Mum looked surprised when I showed her the tattoo later that evening, but she liked it. When Dad accidentally caught a glimpse of it three years later, he too was surprised and tried to rub it off! At this point, I also wrote in my journal:

"These are the things I have learnt, experienced, discovered and are uncovering as I recover: Wisdom, choice, peace, trust, openness, spontaneity, unconditional love, colour, excitement, thankfulness, endurance, hope, self-care, ability to be, freedom, purpose, guidance, grace, deep filling, strength, gentleness, sparks of joy and compassion. I need to hold onto and invest in these. They are of true value and bring life to myself and those I connect with. These are the reasons (and I suspect they will grow as I do) why I want to and can leave anorexia behind. They are real to me and are better than what any surface things of the world offer. They are of light, not darkness."

Then, as springtime neared, I asked Mum, "Do you think we could go on a holiday and a dolphin-watching cruise?" Mum agreed, after all, we had both always wanted to do it. However, a week before our trip, Mum pulled out because of agoraphobia. I felt angry and disappointed. Restricting my eating in the past helped with difficult emotions, but this time I kept eating while acknowledging the truth that Mum deeply valued our relationship, yet just found it too hard to go. What to do with the anger and disappointment? Instead of being angry, I chose to be loving and gracious. I held onto the truth that we are all on a journey of learning, growing and healing, Mum and I included. Feeling disappointed, I drew closer to God, knowing he would meet all my needs. In doing this, my anger further dissipated.

Choosing to be loving and gracious, however, was not an easy feat. To love and be gracious required me to connect with my heart, express it and feel an array of emotions—everything opposite to anorexia. It even meant I may feel love in return. Yet, it was the natural next step to take. Equipped with the truths I was gathering and trusting God, I took this step and found further inner life and restoration—nothing to fear.

After working through my feelings, I went on the holiday alone. I caught a train to the Central Coast. Standing in the carriage all the way (still obviously had an exercise issue to overcome), I read *Victory Over the Darkness* by Neil T. Anderson.[9] I didn't put it down the entire trip. I learnt life-giving truths about myself I had never known before, namely my spiritual identity. For instance, I learnt how I am unconditionally loved. I am a conqueror. I am free of condemnation. I am altogether beautiful. I have a spirit of power and love. I am salt and light to the earth, and I am seated with Jesus in the heavenly realms (John 3:16, 1:12, Romans 8:35-39, 8:1-2, Song of Solomon 4:7, 2 Timothy 1:7, Matthew 5:13-14 and Ephesians 2:6).

Once at the holiday destination, I met up with a friend, and we went on the cruise together, where we saw dolphins splashing carefree in the water. That night, I dined solo in an Italian restaurant by the marina. In typical eating disorder style, I asked the waitress, "What ingredients are in the pasta dish?" Even though I resorted to selecting the meal with the lowest fat content, I ordered something, sat in a restaurant and somewhat enjoyed the new experience. So, in the end, the holiday worked out fine, and I learnt, lived and grew a little more too.

As holidays became less anxiety-provoking and more exciting, I planned more. I flew to tropical Rockhampton in December to visit my stepdad. I valued reconnecting with important people in my life—and he was one of them. We spent Christmas together. With a sense of joy, he could cook up a roast to celebrate.

"Can you cook it without oil?" I asked, well, pleaded.

"A roast has to have oil," he replied, almost in disbelief.

We compromised, and my stepdad cooked it in just a little oil. While visiting, we went to the movies, a crocodile farm and beachside markets—we had fun like old times.

My stepdad lived near Great Keppel Island, so I booked myself a mini holiday there. I caught a boat to the island and was allotted a room with another girl. We went snorkelling over the coral reefs, camel riding along the beach, joined group activities and went to the nightclub together. I had a lot of fun to catch up on! In the evening, I relaxed, read a book by the poolside and sat on the beach under the starlit sky, watching the waves rolling in as I prayed.

The book I read on the island was *Run Baby Run* by Nicky Cruz and Jamie Buckingham.[10] It tells the true story of how God intervened in a young gangster's life and completely turned it around, even when everyone else had given up on him. His story was compelling, and I could relate to aspects of it. On my trip home, I gave the book away to a man I met on the train who was struggling with drug addiction. Growing up, I had an eye to see and a heart to include people who were different or left out, and through my time in psychiatric hospitals, I learnt I could relate to and connect with people of all ages and backgrounds. Nearly recovered, I found myself in a better position to extend the heart of God to others. Life was flowing through me, and it felt good—really good.

Having spent many years in treatment, I had little work experience, so 2006 was the year to do something about it. I enrolled in a waitress and barista course. I volunteered at a youth café and worked part-time door knocking, fundraising for cancer research (the walking side of it suited me well).

I re-enrolled in intercultural studies too. This time I didn't study via distance education, instead I attended the city campus. Sharon's parents lived near the campus and kindly offered to let me stay at their place. It was a helpful offer but also daunting. It meant sharing meals with them and being social. Yet, with the life skills I had gained during treatment, along with my spiritual beliefs, I could face new challenges, knowing that my world would open up a little more each time.

The students at the campus were friendly and included me at their lunch table. Having often been left out of social circles growing up and isolated through anorexia, I cherished being included. I also joined in conversations, which was relieving and enjoyable. In other ways, however, I didn't quite fit in, but it didn't bother me. For instance, unlike other students, I hand-wrote all my assignments. I had missed the leap into the world of laptops and the internet, having been so insulated in anorexia and treatment. And even though I now had the opportunity to catch up with technology, I wasn't interested. I was determined to connect with people and thought technology would be a distraction and a waste of time. I had strong, alternate beliefs, but at least they now aligned with what I valued in life.

Eating and Weight

It wasn't all smooth sailing, though, far from it. There were times I wondered, *Is this ever going to stop? Is every day before me going to present anxiety around food? When will food just be food?* Eating rules, habits and fears had entangled themselves in every aspect of my life, and although I had come far in working through it all, I still had much work to do.

Contending with hunger versus satiety, acting wisely in response, and feeling an array of emotions once again, was a daily challenge. I still watched what I ate, and on the other hand, I secretly grazed on sweet foods and carbs. I ate out with friends, but not without anxiety. I also had little tolerance for feeling hungry, as it reminded me of all the years of starving, yet feeling full was not easy either. I often felt overwhelmed and tired, but no matter how bad I felt any given day, I didn't cut back my intake. I ate like a robot, even if I was unwell. Eating like this was less scary, as I was used to disconnecting from my feelings, and it helped to stop the slippery slope of restricting food types and portion sizes. However, it wasn't ideal. Ideally, I would eat with complete freedom, but this was good for now.

Along with eating challenges, people I had never met before, in little corner stores or who lived three blocks away, commented, "You've gained weight and look really well now." I didn't interpret their comments as "she looks fat." Yet, I did find comments anxiety-provoking, especially as I was still underweight and had more weight to gain. I thought, *If people think I look well now, they'll think I'm fat when I get to my natural weight.* I also felt exposed, with others noticing my body and strangers commenting. And even though it was tempting to think, *If I look fine now, I'll stop right here with normalising my eating and exercise,* I was also acutely aware that if I were to restrict my intake, even slightly, I could find myself trapped once again. So, as difficult as it was hearing weight-related comments, they were never enough to set me back. I had come too far to turn around now.

Activating self-care, being social, staying involved in my studies and church, as well as therapy and prayer, all helped me to manage eating and weight challenges. For instance, one night, feeling overwhelmed, I prayed to God, "Please hold me secure; recovery is hard. I feel scared." The following day, as I rode a rattly old train home from the city, battling eating disorder thoughts, I suddenly felt peace from shoulder to shoulder across my chest. And in that moment, I knew God was holding me secure, giving me the courage and strength I needed to keep pressing on.

Books on positive self-image, like *Captivating* by John and Stasi Eldredge,[11] also encouraged me. Through their book, I discovered how women are uniquely beautiful, inside and out, and that our whole selves, body included, matter to God. It helped redefine beauty for me in a far richer and more appealing way than the simple "beauty comes in all shapes and sizes" message. It spoke to my heart and at just the right time.

By mid-year, for the first time since anorexia, I reached a BMI of 20. I felt very self-conscious that people could see an outward difference in me and that the difference was my weight. Yet, I didn't think I looked fat or ugly, nor did I feel disgusted or distressed. Neither did I feel great. I simply felt okay. I thought it strange, but once I reached my natural weight, guys started to take an interest in me. Seeing my family and friends relieved and happy that I was healthy, reassured me too.

I also saw a dietitian. However, to my detriment, I found it hard to be honest with her about what I ate. I felt ashamed and like I was letting her down by still eating diet food, so I didn't gain the full benefit of her help. I felt more comfortable with my psychologist.

Cheerleader

My psychologist, who I had been seeing for two and a half years, was like a personal cheerleader, celebrating every obstacle I overcame. She pushed me to move beyond things I was struggling with, but with insight, care and skill. Her approach helped me to feel safe and more inclined to share my thoughts, feelings and behaviours. I shared with her how I thought I looked "big" in a recent photograph taken at a wedding. I would have kept this to myself in the past, not wanting to sound vain or have my fears confirmed. Then, throughout anorexia, I became accustomed to people discounting much of what I said as the "eating disorder talking," often making me hesitant to share. Yet, I trusted my psychologist, and to my relief, she simply said, "Bring the photo in and show me." So, I did. Looking at the photo together, she said, "You look amazing, but I can see what you are saying. This photo makes you look bigger than you are. I think it's the angle." And in that moment, my fear, shame and negative self-talk fell silent. I also started looking at myself differently in photos. Letting someone in, the right person, mind you, really did help. She was also a bit alternative. For instance, instead of accepting fees for one appointment, she told me, "I want you to keep the money and buy Christina Aguilera's album and listen to her song *Beautiful*." I liked my psychologist. I respected her and felt supported and overall understood.

Having said that, I didn't tell her I was now experiencing intrusive thoughts and images flashing across my mind, unrelated to the eating disorder but perhaps linked to OCD. I felt ashamed and unsure if she could help anyway, as I believed a spiritual element was at play. When these thoughts or images appeared, I flicked myself or flinched my right shoulder. I hated them. Yet, I didn't feel the need to engage in complex rituals to counteract the disturbing images because I knew I was forgiven and free from condemnation. I also believed they weren't from me. Still, it was unpleasant, and I had experienced enough mental torment over the years, so talking about this would have helped, as well as receiving prayer and Christian counsel.

In another session, my psychologist noted, "It seems like your world grows smaller when you don't spend time with people." She was right. Relationships are so important. So, next on the agenda was making specific efforts to hang out regularly with friends. Like most things, the more I did it, the more natural it became. I enjoyed checking out Tanya's band, watching movies with Fiona and catching up with Dianna and church friends. I was behind on dating, driving and knowing what drink to order at a bar, but they didn't seem to mind. Sharon and I kept up our friendship too. We did healthful things together, like exploring lookouts and ice-skating. We even attended a Buddhist meeting at Newtown one night (my studies included world religions) and often spent time by the river connecting with God. I also joined a few guys from my church in supplying free food and drinks in the local housing commission area. I enjoyed serving people and the friendships I built with them. Having a network of friends now meant a lot to me, more than ever.

Free to Explore

As spring arrived, our church hosted a "Stream of Green" weekend away for young adults. I intended to go only for one day, but with encouragement from my psychologist, I went for the whole three. It meant no exercise for three days and eating whatever was served. It meant doing this while engaging with people and daring to enjoy it all. I went and had a wonderful time! I maintained a structured daily routine and brought some of my own food, but I only struggled once with eating. I had sat down at the dining table but felt overwhelmed, so I walked outside, recalled truths, prayed and then walked back in and ate most of my meal. Spiritually, attending the retreat was also worthwhile. It was here that I felt God's love for the first time. His love felt warm and filled every space of my heart. I knew God loved me, but to feel it was something else.

Afterwards, Pastor Paul invited people to travel with him to Papua New Guinea (PNG) to provide health education and spiritual encouragement to the people, as well as practical love. I was keen to be a part of it. I was also nervous about eating different foods and not exercising for two weeks. Yet, I was up for the challenge, and my psychologist provided support to see it through.

I felt excited. After all the years of anorexia and numbness in my heart, my childhood dream of helping people overseas was coming true. I travelled with a team of four people—we had an amazing time. I thoroughly enjoyed relating with the seaside villagers, being blessed by their generous hospitality, eating cooked bananas and riding in the back of utes while dodging potholes. I even shared at gatherings about my life-changing encounter with supernatural peace. Being new at recovery, I stuck to eating foods I felt comfortable with, struggled with doing no exercise and felt down at times, but I prayed, journaled and kept engaging with the experience, and loved it.

The day after arriving home from PNG, a guy who was a part of the team wanted to hang out with me, and we started dating. He was my first boyfriend at age twenty-five.

I soon discovered that dating also meant eating with someone and eating foods I usually avoided. My boyfriend brought crackers, fancy cheeses and wine over one evening to share. I had never eaten food like this before nor drunk wine. It felt nerve-racking and fun all at once. Then, there were meals he cooked, like satay chicken, which triggered anxiety because they weren't something I allowed myself to eat yet, but I set my mind on truths and ate and enjoyed these meals anyhow. There were others, however, he wanted to cook, like lasagne, that were too anxiety-provoking. I even recall he suggested cooking it while we were out bushwalking. Despite spending hours trekking through the bush, I walked up a steep incline so fast because of the adrenaline rushing through me, thinking, *How am I going to eat lasagne?*

Now that I was in a relationship, spending a lot of time on my own, having days planned out and eating at certain times was also challenged. It felt overwhelming to begin with. Yet, continuing to receive support from my psychologist and spiritual encouragement from the church helped. To my delight, I found for the first time in many years that I could have fun, be silly and laugh uncontrollably. It was also encouraging to hear from my boyfriend that I was attractive. So, I continued down the path of finding and experiencing freedom and life to the fullest.

8. A New Day

Road trips are fun, right? In January 2007, Dad, his new partner, my boyfriend and I packed our cars and headed to South Australia to celebrate my little sister's twenty-first birthday. My boyfriend and I then explored Western Australia, Victoria and Queensland. During our travels, he returned home, and I caught a train on my own to Alice Springs. I journeyed for two days through the outback, with only red dirt and the odd kangaroo in sight. Arriving in Alice, I caught up with my cousin and his young family. I had only seen my cousin a few times growing up, and even though he lived far away, my eating disorder had affected him too. He shared, "I'm not religious or anything, but I prayed for you during your eating disorder, Cas, and I'm so glad you are better."

The trip, although it had highlights, had its difficulties too. While in Alice, I received news that Gran had suddenly passed away, and as I had caught a nasty tummy bug, I couldn't get to her funeral. I didn't cry until I verbalised out loud to my Aunty, who was visiting, "My Gran just died." Then the tears flowed.

"You're allowed to be sad when your Grannie dies," said Aunty while offering a hug.

As our trip continued, there were other challenges to face. I still ate at very rigid set times, which caused tension between my boyfriend and myself. Then, there were the typical and not-so-typical relationship issues to work through. Added to the mix, we visited different churches along our travels. We found they had varying theological teachings, and I got confused and distressed about whether God accepted me all over again. One church taught that if I were indeed a Christian, I would speak in tongues, but I didn't. Another said I needed to be baptised to be guaranteed eternal life, but I hadn't been. In my mind and emotions, I felt pulled in many directions. I tried to be mindful of the spiritual truths I had already found about God's love and who I am to him. I also searched out further truths and read the entire *New Testament* in two days. Through careful reading, I regained confidence that Jesus qualified me to have an eternal relationship with God, and that nothing could add or subtract from this.

Health and Healing

When the travelling was over, keeping my mind on truths continued to help me walk in the freedom I had and was finding. This was especially apparent when my weight increased. I didn't like the weight gain. Yet, with recalling spiritual truths about my identity and dietetic facts on nutrition and weight, self-criticism and fear didn't return. Instead, I could focus on further normalising my eating by adding foods I still avoided and overcoming my grazing habit. I also had ongoing support from my psychologist and trusted that my metabolism would pick up in time and my weight would be fine as long as my eating was.

Considering I had severe anorexia, my body had healed fairly well. I hadn't escaped the disorder unscathed, though. I had fatigue, hypoglycaemia, systemic candida and severe constipation. All these health issues interlinked and influenced my carbohydrate cravings and weight. So, as the year proceeded and my health issues remained, I saw two highly recommended gastro specialists. Neither were of help. One didn't even believe I used to have anorexia until he saw the PEG scar. I persisted, however, in seeking help with my health and saw an allergy specialist. He found I had an extreme dust allergy, which can cause sinusitis and fatigue. Further tests confirmed I had candida in my system. I learnt this could cause fatigue, sugar cravings and sinus too. The solution? To be desensitised against dust, avoid foods with yeast and add coconut oil to my food. It had taken me years to incorporate healthy fats into my daily diet, but now I started to. And to my surprise, my weight didn't go up at all. My allergies also eased. Unfortunately, my fatigue and other health issues weren't readily healed.

Nevertheless, it did feel healing to share my recovery story at a community meeting. Being outdoors, visiting peaceful prayer rooms in the countryside and practising mindfulness brought a sense of wellbeing too. It also felt good to graduate from Tabor College, not with a diploma like I planned, but a Certificate IV. Having learnt all I was interested in, I felt free to stop the degree there. Afterwards, I celebrated with friends at a Thai restaurant, as you do.

Sharing meals with people other than my mum or boyfriend became the new norm. Every Wednesday evening, a small bunch of us from my church gathered around a meal, shared life and encouraged each other spiritually. Even though I still watched what I ate, anxiety didn't rule the situation, nor did eating become the main event. Instead, I enjoyed sharing meals with what felt like a family, learning from others and feeling cared for. It felt nourishing for both my body and soul.

I spent the rest of the year babysitting, delivering papers and volunteering in a children's drop-in centre in the city. The kids at the centre were a sweet and refreshing blessing. Kids don't care about outward appearance. Kindness, showing interest in them and holding their hands is what counts in their eyes.

During this time, I also went on another trip to PNG with my boyfriend, pastor and several other friends from church. We shared at gatherings, made new friends, prayed and offered practical help to people in the hospital and seaside shanties. And once again, I thoroughly enjoyed it.

In the new year, I resolved to get my driver's license. After all, I was almost twenty-seven years old. I had been too unwell to learn when all my friends did, yet now I was ready. Dad was eager to be my driving teacher. He did a fantastic job, and I finally got my L's thanks to him.

I also heard about a nursing traineeship and how this was the last year they would offer it. After all my time spent in hospitals, I didn't want to work in them, but I wanted a skill to take abroad for future ministry in developing countries, so I applied. I wasn't expecting to be accepted to join a class of forty students out of the 400 applicants, but I was. The highest level of math I had completed was to ninth grade (a friend in the adolescent psych unit did most of my tenth grade math, he had OCD and to my advantage, was great with numbers!), so I shouldn't have even scored a place in nursing. The traineeship was full-on. My energy levels were low, my relationship with my boyfriend was rocky and I only studied the night before exams. I had to insert NG tubes and face other situations in the hospital setting that reminded me of anorexia. Yet, I enjoyed the course and graduated with good marks.

Undoubtedly, God opened the door for nursing and saw me through. A pastor from a different church who barely knew me and didn't know about my nursing prophesied over me that year. He said, "I see you driving an ambulance. You are a nurse. The ambulance is full of women and children. You have a gift of mercy; your mercy is the same as that of Jesus."

The following year, in 2009, I graduated as an enrolled nurse. I also finally got baptised. As a child, I believed I needed to be baptised to be a "good" Christian and to receive eternal life, but I have since learnt otherwise. I now understand that baptism is essentially and profoundly an act that helps us identify with being cleansed, forgiven and made new, once and for all, through Jesus' life, death and resurrection. It also serves as an outward declaration to others of one's choice to follow Jesus. Nothing more, nothing less.

To celebrate and contemplate the future, Sharon and I took a mini road trip to the Central Coast. We played in the hotel pool on inflatable toys, relaxed with facials and wine and rose early to catch the sunrise over the bay. We also visited a church together. Here, a pastor I had never met prophesied over me, saying, "I see you going to remote villages and speaking different languages. The words you speak will overflow from your heart and bring transformation." Another lady said, "God is taking you to a new place to protect and establish you; he is doing something new." On returning from our time away, I started looking for nursing jobs around my hometown, but none were available.

I hadn't planned to move, but a couple of months later, I was offered a nursing position in a small coastal country town over 500 km away. I had never heard of this tiny town before and didn't know anyone there. I told myself, *I would only be gone for six months.* I thought relocating would also give my boyfriend and me a fresh perspective on whether to keep seeing each other or end it. Moving felt like an adventure and a much-welcomed change.

Stepping Out

With moving away, my psychology appointments, which had become less frequent, ended. Although I felt fine stepping out on my own, my psychologist assured me I could contact her anytime if needed. Having good friends to share life's ups and downs with now became my primary source of support. Sharon, being one of them, visited with her son the first week of moving. We explored my new surroundings and enjoyed painting on the rock wall by the seaside. We painted a large picture of an eye, with a rainbow for its eyebrow and the blue ocean beneath. On our art piece, we declared we would, "Seek, find and walk out the path of life, and know God's presence, forevermore."

I soon discovered the North Coast of Eastern Australia offers stunning scenery; from secluded beaches and rolling green hills to lush rainforests with spectacular waterfalls and crystal-clear creeks for swimming. I fell in love with it—especially my sunset beach walks, where I easily connected with God. I also joined aqua aerobics and a women's quilting club. I made friends at a local church and received relationship counselling from the pastor's wife. I enjoyed checking out the ever-so-interesting hippy markets and eating at little boutique cafes too.

I lived in the nursing quarters and worked part-time on the hospital's medical ward. Being new at nursing, I found the first few months nerve-racking. I had to be assertive, social and face disapproval from other nurses when I made mistakes. Over time, however, my confidence increased, and I grew to really like my job, staff included.

As the North Coast is known for its alternative lifestyle, it also proved helpful for seeking healing for minor but ongoing health problems post-anorexia. Here, I saw a reflexologist and an iridologist, who both diagnosed me with adrenal exhaustion, which can cause fatigue. I enjoyed buying fresh produce, veggie juices, my first salt lamp and breathing in the country air. Having a kitchen downstairs in the nursing quarters even helped me to cut back on my grazing habit. Cut back, not cure, but I was fine with that—no need to perfect everything. My weight also settled around a BMI of 21.

In no time, the six months were up. I enjoyed my new lifestyle. And my boyfriend and I still hadn't sorted things out, so I told myself, *I'll stay just another six months.*

Sharon and Fiona both visited over the summer. We watched fireworks light up the beach as the New Year began. We also checked out *The Butterfly House*, homegrown fruit stalls, boho cafes and drove my old SAAB through the beautiful, lush green Northern Tablelands. Life was good, but again, not perfect and not without struggles.

Not long into the year, my boyfriend phoned and said he was ending our relationship. We had broken up many times (so much so that Fiona referred to our relationship status as "undefined"), but I was always desperate to get back together. This time, though, was different. I decided I couldn't be his girlfriend unless our relationship improved. Two months later, he wanted to get back together. I explained I couldn't. The problem was, I couldn't completely walk away either. I caused a lot of grief between us, and we drifted in and out of a non-committed, destructive relationship for the rest of the year.

While this was happening, my stepdad was diagnosed with a rare and aggressive cancer on his forehead. The doctor said he may only have weeks to live with it being too advanced for radiotherapy or an operation to be successful. So, I flew to Queensland to visit him. I prayed for my stepdad's healing and asked others to pray too. My stepdad wanted to use his time left to travel through Europe. On return from overseas, to the doctor's amazement, his cancer disappeared, for now.

It was an exceedingly difficult period; keeping in touch with friends helped. In the wintertime, Fiona drove up to celebrate our twenty-ninth birthdays together. We headed out to the beach at dusk and built a campfire near the ocean's shore. We sat, chatted and roasted marshmallows over a crackling fire, one of my favourite things to do. I took along a few journals from the anorexia years. I tore up the pages one by one and dropped them into the fire, watching the flames disintegrate them. I admit, I felt embarrassed that many pages had very messy writing with swear words that could easily be seen, but I trusted that good friends accept you as you are.

Just a week later, someone suggested that I should write a book about my eating disorder experience. Over the years, Sharon and I had discussed what we would like to tell others about recovery. We had even talked of writing a book together someday, but until now, I didn't feel ready to put my past into writing. However, with some of my darkest journals now in ashes, I felt like a new door opened. Ever so slowly, I began jotting down pieces of my story, looking through old cards, finding past medical records and reading other journals I had safely kept while also praying— with the goal of one day publishing a book that would shine hope.

Welcoming in 2011, my big sister and I celebrated our first New Year's Eve together. We played snooker and shared drinks in her beach shack with a couple of her mates. While in South Australia, I also enrolled in summer school. The school was for medical professionals who wanted to gain knowledge and skills to equip them to provide health services to people in developing nations.

On returning home, my boyfriend and I broke up for the last time. I faced the deepest pain, sadness and loss I had ever experienced, the kind that makes you ache inside, and momentarily it feels like the world is standing still. Yet depression, anorexia and OCD didn't arise. When I turned to God, he stepped in. He spoke to me through dreams, brought loving people into my life, gave me peace and the gift of a spiritual language. He also spoke words directly to me and through other people, which built me up and brought healing to deep wounds. I felt him closer than I had ever felt before, not just in my heart but with my whole being. God didn't hold back his love for me, even though I hadn't been putting him first in my life. It's hard to describe the impact, presence and power of God. Simply put, I found God is easily accessible, his Spirit is alive and strong in me, and he knows and cares about my heart like no other. With God, despite my brokenness and sin, I am not left to drown in sorrow—I can dance in the rain.

The same week of the breakup, I heard there was an opening for a Scripture teacher at the local primary school. Though parts of my world felt shattered, my heart to know God and make him known remained protected, and I was keen to get involved. Teaching an entire class of kindergarten students was daunting, yet I absolutely enjoyed it. I loved imparting something good into their lives and seeing their response. In turn, they taught and blessed me much. Their favourite part of the lesson was prayer time. "Thank you, God, for Miss Cassie. Please tell her she is a smart cookie," prayed one precious and ever-so-sweet little girl.

Unexpected blessings continued to come my way. A friend, Hannah, asked me if I'd like to go with some people from her church to a drug and alcohol rehab centre to hang out with and support the residents. I was keen to be a part of it, so Hannah arranged for her brother Aaron to drive me there. A rehab centre is not the most romantic of places to get to know a guy, but somehow, I had caught Aaron's attention. The following day, I received a bold text saying, "You are an AMAZING woman. Can we meet up again?" I felt surprised, delighted and curious. After hanging out with Aaron for a few months, I asked God, "If it's good for Aaron and me to date, can you send him back to my door to ask me to be his girlfriend?"

Within moments, I heard a knock at the door. It was Aaron.

"This may sound strange, but I was wondering if you'd be my girlfriend?"

Without hesitation, I said, "Yes."

To make sure Aaron knew what he was getting himself into before we started dating, I told him, as we sat on a large rock at the beach, all about my past eating disorder and relationship with my first boyfriend. I thought I'd give him a chance to back away before things went any further. My past, however, didn't daunt him, put him off or change how he saw me. Instead, he felt honoured that I was open and honest with him. Did I mention Aaron is also a romantic? He took me for country drives, picnics by waterfalls and lit campfires on the beach at sunrise. He brought all my favourite foods when I was sick, sent flowers to work and told me, "You're beautiful." Sweet huh?

I rented my own place for the first time as well. My home was now amongst green hills and cows. It was a farm shed turned into a granny flat, which was perfect, well, almost. It came with rats, frogs, chilly winter nights (where I wore UGG boots to bed!) and tank water that ran out, but that's all part of the country experience, and I embraced and enjoyed it all. I also completed a rural emergency nursing course that year to build skills for mission work and continued working at the hospital, gaining more confidence as a nurse.

During the spring, I then travelled with a medical team to Timor-Leste for three weeks. This trip was different from my earlier trips to PNG. I felt at peace with eating whatever food they served and not exercising for three weeks. I gained insight and hands-on practice in setting up and running medical checks in rural conditions. My heart felt full and I hoped to do more of this in the future.

To finish the year, I had the best Christmas I've experienced as an adult. Aaron and I celebrated the birth of Jesus with Mum at her home. We enjoyed a traditional roast, laughed at Mum wearing her shirt inside out and back to front at the dining table, exchanged gifts on Christmas Eve and attended church.

The prophecy spoken over me a couple of years ago was coming true. God had taken me to a new place. He was doing something new in my life, and now he was establishing me in this new season too.

As the new year unfolded, I felt a deeper sense of wellbeing and continued to experience inner and physical restoration. I found joy in caring for others at work, teaching scripture and embracing coastal living. Aaron and I continued dating, and I enjoyed time with him, his family and church. I also sustained healthy eating, and at thirty-one years old, I even joined a gym for the first time! My weight remained at its natural set point too. I continued seeing an allergy specialist and persisted in finding solutions to my fatigue. I maintained friendships from my hometown and the new ones I formed. I continued seeking and receiving prayer at different churches and counsel from wise women to help with past and present relationship issues and decision-making. While not without anxiety or sadness, resting in God and practising mindfulness further allowed peace, hope, love and joy to sprout forth during this time of being and rebuilding.

I even found some solid answers to my post-anorexia health problems. A local gastro specialist ran a few tests, which showed I had extremely severe slow transit constipation. He prescribed a low-fibre diet, as opposed to a high-fibre diet that other doctors recommended, to help ease the discomfort. It wasn't a cure. Yet, it felt good to have someone properly investigate it and provide some answers. Another doctor further discovered that I had hypothyroidism, which can cause low mood, a slow metabolism, fatigue, constipation, sensitivity to coldness and weight gain. I may have had it since recovery, but it wasn't diagnosed until now. The same doctor investigated my fatigue. He found I had low iron counts from poor vitamin C absorption, high pyrrole levels (which is common for people who have a family history of mental illness) and high copper levels, all of which can produce symptoms of fatigue, sinus, headaches, low mood and bowel problems. He prescribed thyroxine and high-quality multivitamins for these imbalances. On top of this, another doctor diagnosed me with chronic fatigue and advised pacing myself energy-wise. Finally, the last phase of physical healing had arrived. I only wished more clinicians received training in treating health complications post-anorexia; not only would it save time, money and energy, but it may even prevent some people from relapsing.

Healing within my relationships also continued. I travelled eight hours by train to see Mum every couple of months. At home, we would talk for ages, watch movies, attend church and eat dinner together. It's embarrassing to share, but Mum would even make my bed for me when visiting. I now loved feeling nurtured and spoilt. Like in any relationship, we have moments of conflict and times when we need to say sorry, but these occasions are few and have positive outcomes. With anorexia in the past, tension around mealtimes has thankfully gone. Mum has been a healthy weight for several years now, too, and keeps pressing forward despite hurdles. Restoring our relationship in the aftermath of anorexia has not been an easy feat, and some areas remain a work in progress, but it has all been worthwhile. Mum means the world to me.

As for Dad, he moved to the same town as me later that year, along with his partner and dog, Rex. I had never lived close to Dad before. Nor had I ever had the opportunity to just pop by for a meal, a chat or ask him to fix my car, but now I did.

Although things were good with my parents, sadly, my stepdad wasn't doing well. The cancer had returned. So, I made several trips interstate. I cooked, shopped and cleaned for him. He shared with me he was thankful to be my stepdad, that he was proud of my nursing profession and gave his blessing if Aaron and I should marry in the future. It was heartbreaking to see him alone and so sick at age fifty-nine. This made me even more grateful that I had Dad around, offering the extra support and encouragement I needed.

Living in the Moment

On a lighter note, in January 2013, I took holiday leave and flew to South Australia to finish the international health course. While there, thanks to a boyfriend who spoils me, we enjoyed a hot-air balloon ride over the gorgeous Barossa Valley at sunrise, followed by a champagne breakfast. You may remember when I was eighteen years old and close to dying in the emergency department, I thought to myself, *I haven't yet been on a hot-air balloon ride.* Well, thirteen years later, I had!

To complete this trip, I suggested to my sisters that we spend a weekend away together. We booked a hotel room and enjoyed a couple of days of shopping, laughing, eating gourmet food and discovering that we share the same shoe size and love for olives! We had never done anything like this before; building memories together was so much fun. If I still had anorexia, there is no way I could have wholeheartedly, freely and joyfully participated in the weekend away as I did with the "sisterhood."

Now for a deep breath. On returning from South Australia, I received devastating news. My stepdad's health had rapidly declined, and he was now receiving palliative care at a hospice. I swiftly repacked my bags and drove interstate to be with him. Within two weeks of my arrival, my stepdad, who fathered me well, sadly passed away, aged sixty from brain and lung cancer. In hindsight, I wouldn't have been able to stay by his bedside, immersed in each moment, day and night, while he was in a coma for ten days, had it happened at any point during my eating disorder. I might have sat or perhaps stood by his bedside for brief periods, but my intake would have dropped to compensate for a change in routine and lack of exercise. And chances are, I would have ended up hospitalised afterwards. During recovery, I could have sat by him for ten days, but calculations, stress and rules would have accompanied me. Now, being there, in any state, next to my dying stepdad would be precious and purposeful, but being free of anorexia meant I could actively engage in each cherished moment. I focused when praying over him, openly shared what was on my heart and freely cried many tears. I had the strength to help him 24/7 and the stamina to support Mum over the phone and the man dying in the bed next door. I also felt both teary and glad when I saw his last smile when my childhood friend Paula visited before he slipped into the coma. Being in the moment even allowed me to sense God's divine presence. As I awoke on the 26th of February, at my stepdad's bedside, I saw the words "I will be there soon" appear in a dream-like vision. Before leaving to freshen up for the day, I prayed *The Lord's Prayer* over my stepdad, kissed him goodbye and said, "I love you." Whilst gone, I received a call that he had passed to heaven. I broke down in tears but also felt a solid comfort and peace. Only two days before, Aaron had seen Jesus in a vision, coming to carry my stepdad home, and now he was there, just as the visions foretold. The day after my stepdad left this world, I even treated myself to a facial, massage and nutritious meal at a cafe with his brother and Aaron. I certainly could not have done and felt all this with anorexia tagging along. Never has it hit me so hard how glad I am to be free.

∞

Last but not least, on the 1st of June, standing on a jetty overlooking the town river, Aaron carefully opened a pre-cut cowrie shell with a diamond and ruby studded ring inside and proposed. While dating, I had prayed and listened to God about whether we should marry. I sensed him say it was my choice, but if I were to marry Aaron, it would be very good. And so, my answer, along with a kiss, was "Yes."

Then, as winter set in, I caught the flu twice and was quite sick, causing my appetite and weight to drop. My BMI was now 18, and my thinking was affected. I stood in the supermarket, unable to decide which sauce to buy. I read the contents and nutrition label and compared it with other products. Reading labels didn't help. It only confused me, as I no longer felt compelled to select items with the least fat or calorie content. I ended up choosing the sauce I wanted, but I didn't like how such a simple decision suddenly became so complicated. Did I have ingrained eating disorder thought patterns that were re-activated with my intake decreasing? Or was it genetics that caused my thinking to alter with my weight dropping? Then again, was I experiencing a spiritual attack, or a combination of all the above factors? I am unsure. Yet, what I do know is that because I didn't have self-critical and deceptive thoughts and no gap in my heart to fill because I had real hope, peace, love and joy, I didn't slip back into anorexia. Instead, I could tap into the spiritual truths and dietetic facts I had gathered through recovery and add healthy supplement drinks to my daily intake to replenish my body. As a result, I soon returned to my natural weight and felt better for it.

With the weather warming up, springtime and our awaited wedding day arrived. Do you remember my family and friends I've spoken about throughout my story? Well, Dianna skilfully braided and curled the bridal parties' hair as we sat in Mum's kitchen chatting and enjoying morning tea. Sharon and Fiona made stunning bridesmaids in their elegant purple and blue gowns, with deep pink roses pinned in their hair. Aaron's brother, Dan, and his best mate, Sage, were our loyal groomsmen, suited up and standing by my soon-to-be husband as he waited at the altar. Our nieces looked sweet in pink flower girl dresses with butterfly prints and flowery garlands. Our little nephew was super cute, sporting a grey suit with a bow tie. My beautiful sisters greeted family and friends as they entered the white sandstone chapel. Dad proudly walked me down a classic, red-carpeted aisle to Misty Edwards' song, "Take My Heart." Mum, just as proud with a big smile and tears, watched. Tanya played the guitar throughout the service, and Paul led the ceremony. It felt like a royal, romantic and sacred occasion as I entered marriage with a one-of-a-kind, handsome, loving, sincere, faith-filled and steadfast man.

To wrap it up, in the lead-up to our marriage, a health professional who supported me during anorexia told me she'd had a dream many years ago when I was still very unwell. She said, "I saw you in my dream as recovered, radiant and full of joy on your wedding day." I love it! There are more to dreams—indeed life, than we know.

Life Now

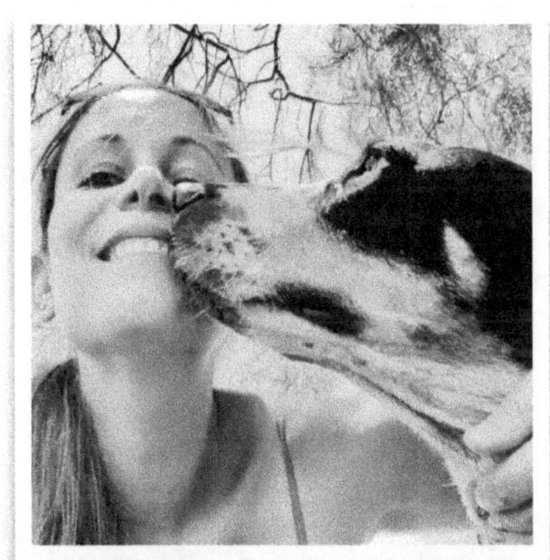

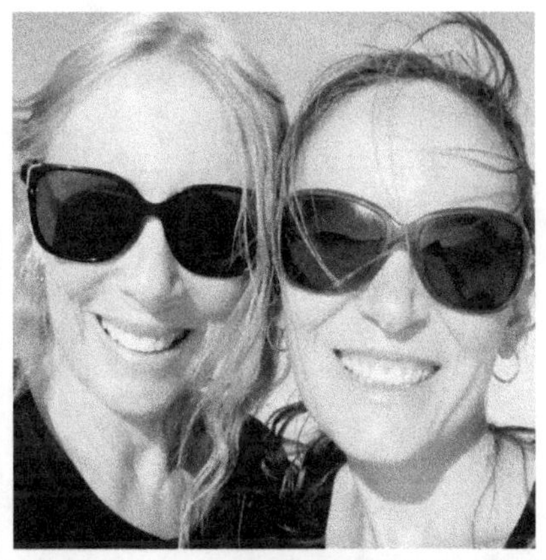

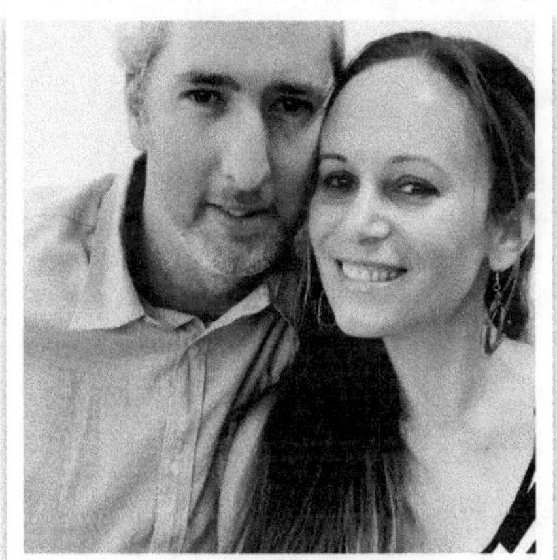

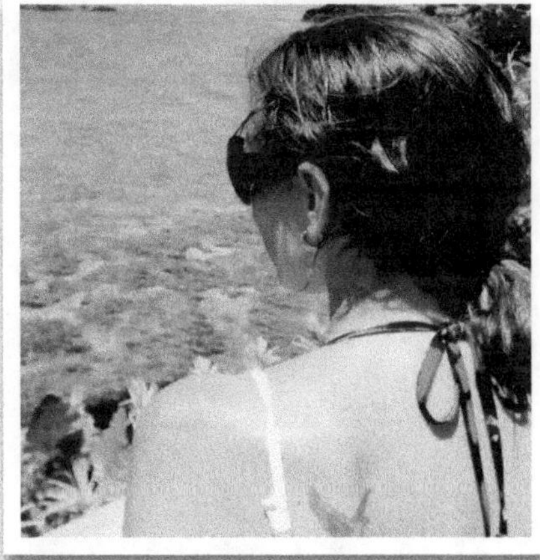

The Ray Collective

A Compilation of Insights and Inspiring Messages

9. Looking Within

I didn't plan to develop anorexia. Who does? All I knew was that I felt angry, sad, hopeless, trapped and hated myself. It also turned out that I had a great deal of determination.

Outwardly, I displayed textbook characteristics of the disorder, such as extreme food restriction, considerable weight loss, persistent behaviour that interfered with weight gain and disturbances in self-image.[12] With these elements combined and genetics thrown into the mix, anorexia unintentionally evolved.

No wonder people perceive it to be a complicated, confusing disorder. However, I believe if we look within, it becomes clearer how anorexia develops and what is needed to overcome it. So, I want to share with you what may be going on internally in the initial stages of the disorder to cultivate a deeper understanding of anorexia, so glimmers of light can start to shine through.

The Hidden Heart

A locket keeps something of value inside.

My heart, drawn to it, goes there to hide.

The chain that holds the locket is made of many links—

a thought, a feeling, a lie, they join together and make me think,

I cannot take this locket off. I will wear it, no matter the cost.

I don't feel happy, pretty or free. I don't like the world set before me.

Somehow, the locket brings relief and numbs my inner grief.

Still void of peace, hope, love and joy, but with my heart encased,

no longer do I feel, and desires are erased.

People at first comment and praise, "The necklace looks good on you."

I am amazed.

It was just a piece of jewellery to wear during the day,

but it offers so much, so at night it will stay.

Consumed, I slowly disappear, and family and friends start to fear,

"You've changed, and it's the necklace we blame.

Take it off. We want the old Cassie again."

But my heart, no one knows, I put inside the locket so long ago.

They do not see; it's not just a matter of taking it off and being me.

If that were the case, I would not have worn it in the first place.

Some try to take it off or advise how, but why should I? What would I be
now?

Just longing for another beautiful chain?

I can't go on; I can't stand this pain.

Then, one day, unexpectedly I find,

the locket opened, my heart touched by the divine.

I hear words that prove true, and links in the chain suddenly undo.

Nothing can contain my heart, now you see,

it's come alive, restored, pumping and free.

The Hidden Heart is a poem based on artwork I did during recovery. It expresses how I felt beyond what others could see. It captures the whole journey through anorexia, yet it also offers unique insight into the initial stages of the disorder.

If you have anorexia, can you relate to aspects of the analogy? Maybe you feel empty within? Consumed by the disorder? Unseen? And yet, you can't let anorexia go?

Still, if you don't have anorexia, perhaps you can also identify with the poem. Has alcohol, money, work, materialism, sexual activity, exercise or even the good old coffee enticed and enslaved you at some point in your life? Such things aren't bad, just like a necklace isn't bad. Yet, addictions can develop if we look to them to regulate our feelings and fulfil needs they were never created to meet. Addictions keep us returning for more, as they only make us feel good temporarily and never address deep issues. All the while—innermost needs remain unmet, and the heart silently suffers. Identity, lifestyle and relationships are often affected too. No matter how big or small, addictions distract and lead us away from truth and knowing life to the fullest.

In many ways, anorexia is like an addiction. Restricting intake and losing weight can feel good at the start and provide relief from "bad" feelings. Yet, in time, the disorder creates anxiety, robs the person of a sense of self, overtakes every part of life and traps them in a harsh world of starvation and fear.

Even if you can't relate to anorexia or an addiction, I suspect you can identify with aspects of how I felt. Have you ever experienced a lack of hope, peace, love or joy? Felt judged by the outside and unseen within?

Trapped and in need of a miracle? If so, you have more in common with someone who has anorexia than you may have ever imagined.

What Starts It All?

The number one question people ask me about anorexia is, "What starts it all?" I suspect many enquire out of sheer curiosity, and that's fine and natural. However, some people want to know how the disorder starts so they can prevent one from taking root or gather clues to help them recover. Others want a deeper understanding of anorexia to support someone through it. So, although there is no single cause for anorexia, from personal experience and listening to others, I believe two dynamics pave the way for the disorder to develop—turmoil and striving.

Turmoil and Striving

I think it's safe to say we all experience inner turmoil at some point. We may feel a multitude of emotions like anxiety, self-hatred, deep depression, intense fear or profound shame. For people with anorexia, awareness of their turmoil and feeling unable to solve it can play a significant role in the disorder starting in the first place.

Then, there is striving, a prevalent feature in our society. It may involve sensing that both oneself and life should and could be better, coupled with the determination to seek that higher standard. However, for those with perfectionist traits and who are highly driven, striving can also pave the way for anorexia.

Even so, turmoil and striving alone do not cause anorexia. However, when linked together, I believe the disorder has the potential to develop. The reason is that striving can be seen as the solution to turmoil. Yet, when striving fails to resolve turmoil, it can grow stronger, leading to more striving, which becomes unhealthy and even harmful.

The Groundwork

Below, I describe the turmoil and striving that laid the groundwork for my disorder to take root. As you read, be mindful this is my experience—everyone is different. And although experiences vary, turmoil and striving remain common dynamics within anorexia and are something that most, if not all, people can relate to in some way or another.

Depression

I spent countless nights crying myself to sleep as a child and into my teens. I felt sad about difficult things within and around me that I felt powerless to change. I also felt "still," the word I used to describe depression as a ten-year-old. Feelings of sadness became familiar and, left unaddressed, increased in the lead up to anorexia.

Social Anxiety

I was at ease with my circle of friends and close family members, but otherwise, I was shy and lacked confidence socially, which I hated. I felt self-conscious standing on my own in social settings or awkwardly trying to join in, time and time again. It caused ongoing anxiety throughout my childhood and in my teens.

Self-Hate

Hate, of inward aspects of myself and then outward, grew. I hated the areas in which I believed I fell below average. For instance, I never aspired to be a perfect daughter, but I thought my attitude towards Mum was far less than acceptable. I never expected to be the most attractive girl at school, but I didn't consider myself attractive at all.

Feeling Unattractive

From a young age, I felt embarrassed about my body, looks and sporting inability, making me very self-conscious. Even though I was a healthy weight, some people considered me overweight by age fourteen, making me feel further ashamed of my appearance. By standards set by society, I deemed myself unattractive. And this mattered; I wanted to feel beautiful, but I didn't.

Loss

Breakups, people moving away, drifting friendships and family members (including pets) passing to heaven, all brought a sense of loss, even grief to my heart as a child and teen. I did my best to manage my feelings, but deep down, sadness remained.

Oppression

I often felt disempowered, unable to voice my thoughts or feelings. For instance, when people made shaming comments about my weight or how much I ate. Repeated episodes like these resulted in the suppression of my emotions, fuelling my depression.

Perfectionism

I persistently thought *I could have done better.* I believed this about school projects, doing my hair, writing on birthday cards, and so on. As a perfectionist, I redid these tasks all over again until I got them right, and even then, it still wasn't good enough.

Anger

Leading into my teens, I felt angry towards people and situations that seemed to block me from what I needed and valued in life. I rarely expressed my anger. Instead, I bottled it up, adding to my depression. Mum was the only person I felt able to express anger with. Yet, not knowing how to view or manage my anger only left me feeling out of control, ashamed and ugly.

Inclusion

I wanted to be liked and accepted, but I didn't always feel this. I saw how people judged others if they fell short of society's ideals and I was sure they applied the same standard of judgment to me. *If I changed aspects of myself*, I thought, *Perhaps people wouldn't judge me and may even get to know, like and include me.*

Religious Beliefs

Growing up, it was important to me to be the best Christian I could. I assumed this involved reading the Bible, praying and loving others. Yet, I struggled to do this, making me think, *I'm not a good Christian*, and I was uncertain if God even loved and accepted me.

Homelife

My parents provided a good upbringing, and I love them dearly, but they are not perfect—no one is. As my parents divorced, I lacked the security and fruit of a healthy marriage. They also struggled with depression, anxiety, perfectionism and poor self-image, which affected my homelife and genetic makeup too.

Trusting in Goals

The message I received from teachers, the media, religion and people I admired was that to succeed and live a fulfilling life, we must strive to be better and push ourselves to achieve. Consequently, I didn't feel at peace within, but fearful. Fearful that I could not function well or achieve much without goals and self-imposed rules.

Why Anorexia?

Perhaps you are now wondering, if factors that lay the groundwork for the disorder have nothing directly to do with food, weight or appearance, why does someone develop anorexia? Although there is still much to learn, drawing on research that says psychological, sociocultural and biological factors contribute to the development of anorexia,[13] together with my experience, I believe there are three main reasons:

1. When turmoil and striving are at work, and someone restricts their intake, whether intentionally or not, anorexia, rather than another type of disorder or addiction can develop.

2. Many people who develop anorexia have self-hate and/or poor body image as their turmoil factors, which can influence someone with perfectionist tendencies to strive for something better and diet in the first place.

3. Lastly, research is looking at how genetics makes someone more likely to lean towards anorexia[14] (my mum had anorexia, so this is very

applicable to me). However, they still recognise that genetics alone do not account for the disorder.

Self-Criticism and Deception

Turmoil and striving can pave the way for anorexia. Yet, in the background, self-criticism and deception are also at work. Self-criticism and deception not only feed the turmoil and striving, but also encourage starvation and fear.

For instance, I recall self-criticism taunting, "You're fat, stupid and ugly," and deception whispering that "Dieting will offer solutions." What sneaky lies! Dieting, taken to the extreme, certainly did not provide solutions, but it did subdue feelings, so turmoil issues *seemed* dealt with. It also proved the ultimate test of pushing myself to the limit, eclipsing the need to strive in other areas. Extreme dieting that led to starvation, however, then locked me into anorexia. With starvation came malnourishment, relentless fatigue, increased interest in food, decreased interest in the outside world, chemical imbalances and the inability to think in big-picture terms. It also affected my critical self-talk, making it fixated on food and weight, which made eating even harder.

All the while, the deeper feelings of turmoil—shame, worthlessness and hopelessness—lingered, and I began believing the condemning lie that *I deserved no better. And, if I dared let anorexia go, a life of turmoil awaited.* So, starving and full of fear, I stayed captive to the disorder and on the brink of death until a way forward presented itself.

Looking back on my journal entries, I can now see how self-criticism and deception influenced my thoughts as I developed anorexia. So, I'm sharing some of my private entries with you because once we learn to identify self-critical and deceptive thoughts, they begin to lose their power. It's like flicking on a light switch and watching the dark scatter.

As you read the entries, can you spot self-criticism and deception in my thinking? Possibly even in your own thought life too?

Sometimes, it's hard to discern what thoughts are critical and deceiving, so talking with someone about them can help. Being mindful that self-criticism and deception never lead to true freedom can also be helpful. So, if your beliefs bring freedom in one area of your life but entrapment in another, you can be sure criticism and deception are at work.

Once we've identified the critical and deceptive thoughts, as I've done for each entry, we can then search out truths to replace the lies—truths that set us free.

June 1996

"I love being outdoors on the cool winter night, camping around the warm blazing fire. I love the stars, clouds and dark blue night sky against the black silhouettes of the trees. There is even a horse in the field tonight. It looks about perfect."

This extract, written at fourteen years old, differs from the rest. It captures a moment of living in the present, feeling wonder and awe, and expressing my heart's delight. When I was a child, I looked at the stars and concluded God must exist, and this felt similar. I sensed something beyond myself, something spiritual and beautiful—before anorexia stepped in.

July 1996

"My face has pimples all over it. I have never had them my whole life, and now they've attacked my face and made me look stupider than I already do. I guess that's life. School sucks this year too. None of my friends are in my classes besides music, which is the only good thing about music. I'm not doing well at school either. I've passed everything, but I could do better. Most of the work is boring and pointless anyway."

Depression was growing, and I was seeing everything through a negative lens. I had acne, but I didn't look stupid (how does someone even look stupid anyway?) So, this was clearly a lie. I was doing okay at school but not as good as usual, and because of my high standards and feeling down, self-criticism also influenced this area of self-perception.

August 1996

"This is my Monday to Friday after school plan: Study 3-4 pm. Dress 4-4:15 pm. Walk the dog 4:15-5 pm. Shower 5-6 pm. Dinner 6-7 pm. Chores 7-8 pm. TV 8-9 pm. Bed 9 pm-7 am."

Turning fifteen this month, I should have been planning a party. Instead, I was devising rigid routines to help me get through each day and achieve goals. The problem is, although they seemed helpful, they robbed me of living in the moment and enjoying each day to the fullest. Not to mention, I couldn't always stick to them anyway. So, with failing to adhere to my plans, self-criticism would grow louder, and a stronger resolve to succeed would follow. With fear ruling, feeling good if I kept my routines and met goals was now replaced by anxiety and torment if I didn't.

September 1996

"I hate myself for being so shy. If I could change three things about myself right now, they would be to look pretty, be confident and good or at least okay at sport, cos I totally suck at it. I must have also put on so much weight this week because Mum wouldn't let me walk home from school, walk the dog or anything. I've been doing my best to eat healthy, but it's hard when she pushes me to eat ice cream and chocolate. Her comments make it sound like I might be turning anorexic. I'm just finally getting healthy and looking after myself."

"I hate myself…" shows self-criticism at work. "I must have put on so much weight…" was not a fact based on evidence or truth. It's not written here, but at this time, I came to believe losing weight would make me feel good, and it did, temporarily. Yet, the very link between weight and depression was deceptive, because the root cause of my depression was never my weight. I also exaggerated the limits Mum placed on my exercise and the food she offered. Mum occasionally asked if I'd like some ice cream or chocolate, but she didn't push it. I knew she was concerned, but with fear and starvation taking hold, sticking to my goals was all that mattered.

October 1996

"I walked to Hollie's house. I then walked to work, served food all day and walked home afterwards. I ate way too much. Tomorrow, eat less (feel sick) and go for a long walk (post a letter)."

Food became my everything, whether served to others, eaten alone, thought of all day or written about. Likewise, walking each day became my number one priority. Starvation was harsh, so any food eaten, no matter how minimal, tasted incredibly good and felt momentarily comforting. At the same time, criticism and deception meant no matter how little I ate, it was still too much. Writing about food and exercise rather than the time spent with my friend now seemed more important too. Starvation was taking over, my perspective was shifting and my values of friendship and honesty were discounted. My world was turning upside down, but like someone with an addiction, all I thought about was the next meal.

November 1996

"I laughed yesterday in class, the first time I've laughed in months."

Nothing much made me happy anymore. I didn't think that was important, but I was deceived. Although I had stopped feeling happy and carefree before dieting, it worsened with anorexia. Unresolved inner turmoil and the effects of starvation now deprived me of the simple gift of laughter. This is significant because, without joy, we are not fully living.

December 1996

"I feel and look so very fat. At Christmas, I ate a whole baked dinner, salad, pudding, fruit and fizzy drink at lunch. And did no exercise. For the rest of the holidays—cut back my intake, cleanse my skin nightly, study math and science, practise and practise playing the piano, read the whole Bible and be a better daughter and Christian. Get fit, do aerobics, ice-skate, rollerblade and garden. See friends, but no sleepovers."

"I feel and look so very fat," wasn't the truth. Fat is not a feeling, and I looked underweight. It's also healthy and good to enjoy Christmas food, but I only felt anxious with each serving placed before me and guilty for eating, falsely believing I needed more self-control. My proactive plan, therefore, aimed to produce self-discipline and promised to make me feel and be a better person. I didn't see it, but a negative voice was devising my plan. Deception was also at work. I didn't need to achieve goals to feel or be better. I needed to renew my thinking and have my innermost needs met. Yet, I knew none the better, and fear would keep it that way.

January 1997

"Yesterday, because of work and life in general, I came home and cried
myself to sleep. Today was okay though, bearable."

I never blamed starvation for its devastating impact on my life. Instead,
I held "work and life in general" responsible. Starvation, of course, was
the symptom, not the cause of my turmoil and striving. But like an out-
of-control fire that creates its own weather system, including destructive
storms, so too did starvation. I had gone from wanting to live life to the
fullest to accepting bearable living. Starvation had once promised to make
life better, but the truth is, life was slipping away.

February 1997

"I hate myself for not being the Christian I want to be. I hate myself for
being terrible to Mum. I hate myself for not being able to concentrate on
homework. I hate how Jessie died. And I hate that my stepdad is unwell."

I found a way to deal with extreme emotions that kept me going and
didn't lead to suicide. Self-punishment through starvation and excessive
exercise brought relief from self-hate. Counteracting depression through
starvation offered a reprieve from numbness, as feeling hungry was better
than not feeling at all. Yet, do this long enough and starving feels comforting, no longer punishing or uncomfortable. So, what to do with the
hate and depression? Deception insists, "There is no way out." Condemnation adds, "You're not worth it, anyway." Yet neither is true.

March 1997

"Went to outpatients today, lost half a kilo. It's so easy to lose weight. They said I needed to gain weight or else they'd admit me to the hospital. I've been trying hard to put it on. I've been eating a lot. Everyone—and I mean everyone—is saying I'm anorexic. But I'm not. They caught me just in time."

I was eating more and believed it would cause weight gain. Yet, the truth was, I was not trying hard to gain weight, and I was not eating a lot. I focused on and magnified the finer details without seeing the bigger picture. I was under the effects of starvation and didn't know it. I felt free, however, of hating my weight and free from constraints in my life. I also felt empowered that I could overcome obstacles. This was only a counterfeit of freedom and empowerment, as I had fallen into the trap of anorexia. Deep down—I was not free at all.

10. Finding Hope

People often say, "There is hope" concerning recovery. Yet, during severe anorexia, nothing scared me more than the idea of recovery. Instead, I needed a powerful hope. Hope that my soul could find what it longed for and life could prove worth living. I wasn't expecting to discover a hope like this, but thank goodness I did!

If you have anorexia, I understand how it feels to be scarcely surviving while being held captive to fear, so I want you to know there is hope—a life-giving hope. For those supporting someone with anorexia, you, too, undoubtedly need hope. It can be incredibly challenging to watch a person struggle with this disorder. But with hope, you can nourish your soul and maintain the stamina to offer support.

Searching out what our soul longs for and the path to life, however, is a sacred journey that we cannot and should not box. With that in mind, I have written *Finding Hope* to simply offer insight and encouragement if you choose to explore or support this bright alternative avenue for yourself.

Soul Needs

Underneath the surface, people who develop anorexia have significant soul (emotional and mental) needs that are going unmet. Maxine Vorster, who recovered from an eating disorder, also speaks about this in her book *Hidden Hunger*.[15] In fact, turmoil and striving indicate the need for deep peace, hope, love and joy. Self-criticism and deception, likewise, signal the need for life-giving truths. So, how do we find what our soul needs?

If we investigate spirituality, we will find various paths to explore. For myself, my spiritual journey led me to discover how humanity once lived in perfect union with the perfect God. I further learnt that we broke this union, and all perfection, including transcendent hope, peace, love and joy, fell away. Yet, deep down, our soul, even subconsciously, still longs for this. The good news is, however, I also found God has never stopped caring about us and can still supply what our soul needs.

Growing up, depending on my circumstances and how I felt, I had some hope, peace, love and joy. Yet, it was never enough. I longed for something more. Then, amidst severe anorexia, I met God for the first time. Until that point, he was a concept, a belief. Through encountering him, however, I experienced a divine peace that ran deeper than my disorder and supplied what my soul truly longed for. With this, hope appeared, and turmoil and striving unravelled. As I learnt truths about God and who I am, self-criticism and deception also lost their grip. Finally, I had a powerful motive and a means to recover.

And I am not alone. Many people who have explored spirituality have also found hope through awareness of God's presence and his ability to help. For instance, I read how a lady receiving support for an eating disorder said God gave her an inner hope she had never known. Others also expressed finding hope in knowing a God who cares for them and supports their recovery journey.[16]

Perhaps you are now wondering, *Does someone need to encounter God to recover?* No, not necessarily. Many have courageously recovered and are yet to or are still exploring spirituality. Life is an incredible journey, and we can come to know God at any stage. However, I believe he is revealing himself to us, and whoever keeps seeking God will find him and the inner life he brings. With this, recovery from the roots up can also be found.

So, let's look at some turmoil and striving dynamics and how they show that the soul needs something more. By doing this, we see how a life-altering opportunity of seeking what or who can satisfy our deepest longings can present itself. If we walk the spiritual path, we may even find anorexia is no longer needed—because the soul has found what it genuinely longs for.

Uncovering the Spiritual Path

Depression

Emptiness, numbness, fatigue, prolonged sadness and hopelessness are just some words that come to mind when describing depression. People may feel like this for varied and valid reasons. These reasons need exploring and addressing to help the depression. Medication and nutritional restoration are sometimes required too. From experience, this is when people can also encounter authentic peace and hope, even joy. Many fill their days, often unknowingly, with distractions and things that make them feel temporarily good. Someone with depression, however, has reached the point where they need something more. They have come to the end of themselves. Coming to the end of oneself presents a sacred opportunity to seek, cry out and find who or what truly calms, satisfies and uplifts one's soul.

Fear of Adulthood

Some people with anorexia fear adulthood. They may fear transitioning into a womanly or manly body, facing greater expectations, change, growing older and dying or other aspects of being an adult. Their fear, while not always, can stem from past/present abuse, making it very real and not to be taken lightly. Altering their body shape through starvation may delay puberty and help them feel small again. It may be a means of deterring attention from the opposite sex and suppressing feelings of sexual attraction. Or it may slow the process of entering the unknown adult world where responsibilities and sometimes hardships increase.

Looking closer, however, we might find that the fear of adulthood echoes a profound awareness that all is not right and that the soul isn't at peace. Perhaps a longing for restored innocence, affirmation, security, hope and unconditional love resounds within. If we explore the spiritual path, it may even reveal that these needs speak of who we are and who God is, and provide a tangible and safe way to fulfill them. With this, adulthood has the potential to look much brighter and can become something to embrace, not fear.

Anxiety

On the surface, anxiety says, "I feel overwhelmed and uneasy. I must avoid or somehow fix the situation that makes me feel this way." Physical symptoms like shortness of breath, increased heart rate and nausea may also follow. Being anxious about eating, socialising, the unknown, change and so forth is draining, debilitating and unpleasant.

Yet, looking deeper, we can see that anxiety flags the truth that the soul needs to feel centred, at peace, secure and hopeful, while the body needs rebalancing too.

So, someone who acknowledges their anxiety not only has the opportunity to speak to someone about how they feel and to seek treatment for any imbalances that may exist, but they can also find what their soul truly needs.

If they pause and ask God for help, they may encounter a peace that surpasses their unrest and gently restores mental, emotional and even physical health. Placing their trust in God and coming under the shelter of his wings, renewed hope and freedom to live in the present may also appear.

Control

They often say, "People with anorexia feel they have little control over their lives." The world around them and their desires and emotions may feel scary, messy and overwhelming. Feeling life is out of control, they might find refuge, even subconsciously, in controlling the one thing they can—their intake, and consequently weight.

For instance, someone with anorexia may hate aspects of themselves but feel unable to control or change what they hate, apart from their weight. They may even believe they need more self-control and punish themselves through starvation to achieve this. Then again, someone who builds their own constrictive world might be trying to escape from feeling trapped or controlled by other people, and/or society. Not to mention, once malnutrition sets in, the disorder itself takes control. So, while control may appear to be the main issue, underneath it all, similar to anxiety, a profound need for peace, protection, empowerment and freedom exists.

The beauty in this is that these needs resonate within, and so does the desire to have them met. Through listening to these needs and exploring spirituality, we may find a God who is ultimately in control—yet not controlling—and who can help us cultivate healthy self-control too. With this, peace, security, empowerment and freedom, a reality many long to know, can more readily be found.

N.B. The above writings on depression, fear, anxiety and control, as with all the writings within *Beautiful Light,* are not written from a medical professional point of view. Instead, I share my understanding as someone with lived experience of anorexia. So, if you are struggling with any of these, for further help, please see a well-trained medical professional.

Hope, Peace, Love & Joy

Sitting in group therapy, I relayed how an incredible peace swept through me during anorexia and took my underlying depression away. A young woman, also struggling with an eating disorder, piped up, "I want that. Where do I get it from?"

She was hungry for something more. So, if you identify with her or are simply curious about life-giving hope, peace, love and joy, I have some inspiring insights for you! And just like no two recovery stories are alike, neither are people's spiritual experiences. So, along with these insights, I have gathered short stories from friends in Australia and abroad who have also experienced profound hope, peace, love and joy, which I'd love to share with you.

Hope

Hope from God, whether it comes directly or through others, brings assurance that we are never alone—that he is with us and can restore our souls and supply our daily needs. This life-giving hope runs deep. It can also transcend darkness and create a way forward where there seems to be none, making it both accessible and unique.

Christie and Michael's Story

"Many years ago, a friend and mentor said to me, 'In times of grief and confusion, when a person loses hope, we can hope for them.'

I experienced the unshakeable truth of his words on one unforgettable day. Michael, my husband, had hit rock bottom in depression. I stood beside him as he lay in the foetal position on our bed, saying the heartbreaking words, 'I have no hope left.' Instantly, deep peace replaced the anguish I had been feeling for years and the words 'I will hope for you' poured out of me. I knew the Holy Spirit was speaking through me with clarity and confidence. The following day, the heaviness that had settled on my husband for years lifted.

The transformation in him over the next few months was profound. I cry every time I think of it. I am so grateful for those words that my friend spoke to me all those years earlier, which at the time were puzzling but became so powerful in a moment of desperation.

It has become a great comfort that as individuals and in community, we can hold on to hope for each other in times of hopelessness."

Peace

Amidst severe anorexia encased in deep depression, I discovered that God's peace perfectly comforts and centres the soul. We don't need to have our acts together or to detach from the pain within and around to find it. This peace is simply a gift from above. As we walk the spiritual path, I also find that inner peace can increase deeper and wider with each new season.

Maria's Story

"Since 2018, my life has been a bit of a rollercoaster, punctuated by the life-threatening diagnosis of my then-partner, three years of working myself into burnout, the shock of infidelity, divorce, the final tearing apart of my family, and helping my children cope with adjustment as their father moved in with the other woman, had a baby with her and married her within a year.

But the peace of God was my protection throughout so many unthinkable, shocking moments of betrayal, loss, and pain. Even through depression, anxiety, and fear, and as I worked through deep-rooted hidden trauma, peace remained. I couldn't always sense or feel it when I wanted to, but it was an unshakable fact in my soul, as true as the daily sunrise.

I never thought one could feel undergirded by the surpassing peace of God while seated in a lawyer's office, proceeding with filing for divorce, with the man whom I'd been married to for nearly thirteen years, sitting next to me, now a stranger. But I did.

The moments when my daughter asks me questions, God provides the words for me to answer her. The moments where my heart wants to break for my children's pain and where I feel like no amount of coping skills, reassurance, or comfort will ever compensate; those moments are the ones where the Spirit reminds me that He gave me peace, He rescued me. He vindicated me out of a situation that was impossible, toxic, and life-draining. And that same peace surrounds my children, sustaining them with a joy I hadn't thought possible.

The peace of God that surpasses understanding is a reality, even amidst suffering. His hands held mine when I wanted out. His tears mingled with mine when I couldn't stop weeping. When I was trying to avoid worrying about my children while they were away, He gave me a vivid vision. The vision was of Jesus walking with my children, His arms around each of them, every time I dropped them off, and received them coming home. This is the hope and peace that sustains me from day to day.

His mercies are new every morning, if I will but take a moment to receive them, take hold of them, and let go of all I want to control to avoid more pain. His peace healed me and continues healing me, moment by moment, conversation by conversation, night by night, and day by day. I am learning to actively choose to live in it, to be intentional in turning to His peace for sustaining strength. And He is there.

His peace is enough to overcome my rage and anger at injustice. His peace brings rest when frustration threatens to consume my mind. His peace comforts me when I have poured out my heart and tears before Him. The most moving truth of it all is that I am safe in it. Learning that is saving and changing my life."

Love

Love is a universal need for all of humankind. Without it, fear and destruction rule. Ironically, however, I feared love during anorexia. Yet, as I came to know God, I found his love to be safe. It nourishes, protects, restores and sustains life. No other love compares to this.

Sharon's Story

"Like pouring cool water on sunburn, letting love in hurt, not because love was painful, it's not, but because it exposed the ache of how I'd been thirsty for love for so long. When I had kept love out, believing I didn't need it, I could avoid these deeper wounds.

Yet, six years into recovery from anorexia, with a good counsellor, I knew I needed to face this topic of love.

I wrestled with it. I didn't feel lovable. I didn't feel important or worthy of people's time and attention, let alone their love. Life had taught me not to trust people to be reliably loving. I reached out for help, but I seemed too complicated, my company too uncomfortable or my needs too needy.

However, I knew that there was a God who was reliably loving, at least to others.

Then, one day, I had a lightbulb moment. I had thought, *God couldn't love me because of how I was*, but I suddenly realised, *I had it the wrong way around*. Believing God couldn't love me because of me wasn't a reflection of me but of God and his ability to love. It seemed like he was saying, 'You're thinking too small about my ability to love. You're thinking less of me than what I truly am.' It helped so much. I didn't have to think better of myself to solve the problem. Instead, I had to think more highly of God. His love is so great that he loves me, just as I am. God can love, and he chooses to. This love was available to me. A love so great that my self-perception was irrelevant. I didn't have to try to figure out an accurate perception of myself. I just had to let love in.

But that pain—when I contemplated this true love, there was an ache inside where love had never been. And I saw it and felt it more than ever.

Yet, I trusted God and little by little, I let his love in.

What did his love feel like? I don't know. I'm not good at just feeling things like feeling loved. What even is that?! Instead, I need love to be tangible, and God's love was. The scriptures paint a picture of love, 'Love is patient, love is kind…' (1 Corinthians 13:4-8). And yes, God has been patient—he has never hurried me to get better before I'm ready to. He knows all the steps that need to take place in my recovery journey and that it will take time. Yes, he has been kind—I see his kindness in the many times and ways he has provided for me. One time, it was a gift of money, just the financial support I needed. Another time, it was a ticket to a Christian conference, just the encouragement I needed. The gifts came through people, but in such a way that I knew they were also from the hand of God. So, I can see God has been and continues to be reliably and unconditionally loving towards me, like no other."

Joy

During anorexia, I found that God gives us joy—his joy. And unlike happiness, inner joy doesn't require us to feel good to experience it. This does not mean that it interrupts our times of grief or dismisses our sorrow, but rather his joy is not overcome by pain and can be accessed even in the midst of it.

Paula's Story

"I decided to follow Jesus when I was seventeen years old. Despite loving and following him, I struggled with anxiety for many years. This anxiety often debilitated me. It impacted my physical and mental health and relationships too. In my early twenties, my boyfriend and I were at a youth conference and were part of the leadership team. For much of the weekend, I felt consumed by anxiety and fear.

Before one meeting, the team gathered to pray. God's presence was very tangible, and as we prayed, the Spirit of God fell on people in different ways. My boyfriend was so overcome by God's presence that he laid almost unconscious for over an hour. When people began to leave the room, my boyfriend remained, unable to physically move. As I reached out to touch him to see if he was okay, the presence of God fell on me, and I began to laugh and laugh and laugh. I laughed until my stomach hurt. It was a different type of laughter to my natural laugh. It came from deep within. It was an unexplainable joy.

That encounter changed something in me. It began to break the anxiety and fear I had lived with for so long. The healing didn't happen all at once. Rather, over the years, I have experienced joy from God on many occasions, bringing more freedom each time.

I am now fifty-four years old, and people often say they love my laughter and see me as joyful. I once read by theologian Henri Nouwen that 'We have to choose joy and keep choosing it every day.' So, when I am not experiencing joy—I remind myself to see or find the joy. And walking with Jesus, I can see it, and I can find it."

N.B. I have two friends named Paula! A different Paula wrote this story about joy than the one mentioned in *Cassandra's Story.*

Endless Encounters

If I heard of someone finding hope through a spiritual encounter, I'd be curious to know if it was a once off. Do they have more to share? Does God still intervene, even when life looks brighter? Essentially, I'd be wondering—*is God real, and can I trust him to sustain my soul?*

So, if you have similar questions, I have a handful of my ongoing spiritual encounters to share with you to offer encouragement that help and hope are available on the road ahead. Not to mention, encountering God is exciting and exciting things are fun to share!

Prophetic Vision

Laying on my bed during early recovery, all I could envision for the future was a constant battle with food, weight and exercise. It felt heavy, overwhelming and depressing. Closing my eyes, in a daydream-like vision, a black knight riding a large, strong, black horse appeared. The following evening, after church, I hung out with a group of young people. We chatted and shared about our week. I didn't tell anyone about my vision of the horse and knight. Yet prophetically, a friend spoke up and said, "Cassie, I see a black knight on a black horse, the spirit of death near you." She then prayed against it. I felt amazed and undone all in one go. My faith and hope arose, and my soul felt intensely cared for as I realised, *We are not alone in our battles. Even once we recover, God is there and able to protect our souls and keep us safe.*

White Light

Fast asleep one night, a bright white light came over me. The light seemed alive and came in waves in a dancing manner. I felt apprehensive. I didn't know what was going on. I then realised—*This must be the Holy Spirit or an angel.* In awe, I continued to experience this all-encompassing, energy-filled light. Then, suddenly, it left. Automatically, with no thought process behind it, I got up, kneeled beside my bed, and prayed for my pregnant friend, who was on a mission trip in Myanmar. In the morning, when I awoke and recalled the night's events, I thought, *Wow, that was amazing but strange.* I hadn't recently thought of my friend, and I rarely prayed kneeling beside my bed and never during the night. Once she returned from overseas, I shared my encounter with her. She said, "Around the time you prayed, I had to leave the village I was staying in because it was becoming dangerous."

I don't know what I prayed that night, but God protected my friend, and my heart was left beating with awe and delight that God would reach out to me to intercede for his daughter and her unborn child. I also felt inspired by the power of prayer and how God intervenes and helps us in ways we may not even see or understand.

Singing and Strings

Laying on my futon sofa, resting in my body but struggling with lust, I set my thoughts on Jesus. As I did, I heard singing. It was Jesus singing. I knew this was a sacred moment. I wasn't asleep or dreaming. I merely had my eyes closed, relaxing. I took special note of all I heard. I heard the song in my right ear. Exquisite stringed instruments played, and I audibly heard a male sing. His voice sounded like he was around thirty years old. I hadn't heard this voice before. It didn't sound angelic. Rather, it sounded like a typical male solo singer's voice, the type that plays the guitar and sings original songs for intimate audiences. His voice was full of sincerity and mellow. As I listened, I heard him sing, "You're holy, holy, holy. I love you, I love you, I have always loved you. I have great plans for you, I have great plans for you, I have great plans for you." I reasoned what I heard, and as I did, the singing and strings stopped. Amazed, I got up and wrote down what had just happened. I felt deeply cherished and blown away by encountering God in such a beautiful way. What's more, I felt encouraged that regardless of what we are struggling with, God reaches out to us with unconditional love, speaking words of life and reminding us of who we are to him.

Spiritual Language

Sitting on my bed, sipping a glass of wine while reading the Bible, I paused and prayed. I don't recall what I prayed apart from, "Please forgive me for not always honouring my parents." Then, although I hadn't asked for the gift of tongues, though I had in the past, I received it. In a split second, I knew I could speak it, and as I spoke, the spiritual language poured out. You may recall I was drinking wine in the lead up to this—but I wasn't drunk! Ever since that night, I have been able to speak in tongues whenever I desire, without fail. Whether I feel fine or am struggling or feel close to God or far, I can always speak it. When I pray in tongues, it helps me to draw closer to him and brings added assurance of his existence and that he is at work today. It also helps me sense what God is saying or doing because I am not using the reasoning part of my mind but relaxing in the Spirit when conversing with him (which is especially helpful when feeling down, anxious or tired). It's a gift that constantly encourages me that God's Spirit lives within, and whether or not we speak in tongues, that the Spirit actively helps us to connect with God, offering peace and refreshment each new day.

N.B. Tongues is the Christian term to describe a spiritually empowered language. It may enable someone to speak a foreign language, such as Italian or Hindi. Tongues can also be a heavenly language. The person, when speaking, has control over their mind and can freely choose when to start and stop talking in tongues. Yet, unless there is an interpreter, mysteriously, they don't know what they are saying, but God does
(Acts 2:4, 6-11, 1 Corinthians 14:2).

Physical Healing

As a nurse, I was looking after a patient who consistently had a high level of pain, no matter how much pain relief we gave him. He was dying. He had no peace or visitors; I felt sad for him.

One evening, I asked, "On a scale of zero to ten, with zero being no pain and ten being severe pain, what score would you rate your pain?"

Like always, he replied, "Ten."

I then took his blood pressure, and while I had my hand on him, counting his pulse, I silently prayed and asked God to take away this man's pain.

A few moments later, I asked, "What is your pain score now?"

He immediately sat up, and with eyes wide opened, he looked stunned. He touched different parts of his body, saying, "I have no pain. I can't believe it. I don't know how, but I have no pain."

He seemed surprised, and I felt elated. I was also moved by who God is and who we are to him. It reminded me that God is near, wanting to help each of us, and although he can personally intervene, he invites us to join him in bringing healing and light to one another.

A Message

Dating Aaron, I shared with him, as we walked barefooted along the seaside, how I talk with God at the beach and find cowrie shells when I sense him speak in return. As I finished sharing, we discovered over ten cowries, all washed up in the same spot. It felt like God was being playful with us. Joining in the playfulness, I explained, "It's traditional for PNG men to buy their wives with cowrie shells," and so began our game of seeking cowries.

Months passed, and I then had a dream. I dreamt Aaron gave me a cowrie. The shell opened, and inside was a pair of ruby earrings. Unsure of what my dream meant, I soon forgot about it. A year later, standing on an old jetty overlooking the town river, Aaron handed me a cowrie shell. He opened it, and inside was a ruby studded ring. After proposing, he said, "If it's not your style, we can remodel the ring into earrings and choose another one together." My dream came true! But there's more. Little did we know that sitting in the chapel on our big day, Pastor Paul would pull out a golden cowrie and centre his talk around it. Paul didn't know our history with cowries—so I listened with delight as he explained how valuable these shells are. "On the outside," he said, "They may have sand on them and become weathered, but it doesn't change their worth." He exhorted us to see the true value that lies within one another and encouraged us that "With a bit of love and care, the shells can polish up and shine anew." Paul's message felt like it was straight from God, one that he orchestrated for us to hear, connect with and recall throughout our marriage.

So, no matter where I am in life, whether strolling down the beach or starting a new chapter, I find comfort and hope in knowing God continues to speak to us and offers guidance—not just through the difficult times but the good times too.

11. Holistic Recovery

Discovering life-giving hope empowered me to step onto the path towards recovery. Yet, it took professional and caring support, spirituality and time for holistic recovery to emerge.

For me, holistic recovery means freedom and health for my body and soul. I no longer feel dominated by the turmoil, striving, self-criticism and deception that was once linked to my eating, exercise and self-perception. I can also freely eat, rest, exercise and maintain a healthy weight. It further indicates that inner restoration, even transformation, has begun.

Moving forward, however, looks different to everyone. It can also involve small and slow steps and what may seem like backward steps. Even so, on a body, soul and spirit level, there remain common threads along the path of recovery.

So, I am keen to share with you what good support that promotes holistic recovery can look like and how spirituality can continue to light the way forward. I hope this offers you further insight and inspiration on your courageous journey ahead.

Effective Professional Support

Professional support helped me to survive anorexia and to restore my health. It also imparted lifelong skills to manage thoughts and emotions constructively. And while it often lacked in providing spiritual care, I believe we can change this. So, let's explore what effective professional support can look like.

The Whole Person

During a therapy session, I was told, "Just leave God out of the picture for now." Instantly, I shut down. Separating spirituality from my thoughts and emotions and how it affected my eating felt impossible. So, before exploring professional support any further, I'd like to highlight how anorexia impacts the whole of a person. I hope this provides insight into how a holistic approach is essential to help and honour people with the disorder.

- Anorexia is a life-threatening disorder. It claims more lives than any other mental illness through the effects of starvation on the body. Even when life is not in immediate danger, anorexia is still damaging the body. Electrolyte imbalances, hair loss, decrease in bone density, disruption of menstrual cycles, intolerance to cold and dizziness are some signs of this. Suicide is also high among people with anorexia.[17]

- Physically, starvation further impacts emotions and thinking processes and heightens eating disorder behaviours, such as cutting food into small pieces, eating slowly and so on.

- Mentally, people with the disorder often struggle to allow themselves to eat everyday foods and in healthy amounts. Many also battle to rest and not over-exercise.

- On top of this, physical and mental comorbidities within anorexia are frequent, such as self-harming, substance abuse, diabetes, coeliac disease, OCD and dissociative disorder.

- Emotionally, people with anorexia may feel bound by deep depression, shame, self-hate, worthlessness, anger, anxiety and fear. They may also suffer from past or present abuse and the trauma it brings.

- Many also seek self-control over their emotions and desires. And self-discipline to achieve their absolute best in several, if not all, areas of life.

- Likewise, for many, anorexia becomes a mechanism to deal with the aspects in the fifth and sixth points above. By remaining underweight, restricting intake and being governed by rules, temporary relief from extreme feelings and a sense of control is found.

- Turmoil, striving, starvation and fear (perhaps even genetics) *significantly* interlink, leaving the person physically, mentally and emotionally entrapped in the disorder.

- Lastly, as the body, soul and spirit intrinsically connect, spiritual beliefs can filter into every aspect of anorexia, offering hope for freedom or fuel for the disorder, depending on the beliefs.[18]

The Team

Building on a whole person approach to treatment, I believe, and research shows, that effective treatment is founded on a team of professionals who have a thorough understanding of anorexia—on a physical, mental, emotional, and ideally, spiritual level. The team may include doctors, nurses, dietitians, physiotherapists, occupational therapists, psychologists, chaplains and others. They skilfully impart helpful strategies to the person with anorexia to help them regain health and freedom while safeguarding their wellbeing. Importantly, the team is non-judgmental, affirming, consistent, compassionate and thinks outside the box. They believe recovery is possible, realise it takes time and that ongoing support is crucial. The team is also patient-centred and works with the person to discern the best level of care for them. Lastly, they involve the family of the person with anorexia and offer them support and guidance too.[19]

Helpful Treatment

Treatment has evolved over the years. Some facilities where I received treatment are now closed, and exciting new ones have opened in Australia, like residential recovery centres. However, many aspects of treatment remain the same. Having experienced multiple treatment settings, I want to share what I found to be the most helpful interventions in promoting physical, mental and emotional health. If you have anorexia or are a caregiver, I hope this informs and reassures you about the effective treatment available. For health professionals, by providing a patient's perspective, I hope you gain new ideas and fresh inspiration.

Individual Therapy

Seeing a psychologist trained in eating disorders with the right personality and skillset was immensely helpful during inpatient and outpatient treatment. My psychologist helped me to feel cared for and supported—wherever I was on my journey. She created a safe place to share thoughts, feelings and behaviours while offering honest feedback and encouragement. We set recovery goals together, and I was encouraged to tap into my spiritual beliefs to achieve them. With individual therapy, I also discovered effective techniques to manage thoughts and emotions. My psychologist also liaised with the eating disorder team to provide a consistent and holistic approach to treatment and offered support for as long as I needed.

Cognitive Behavioural Therapy (CBT)

Using CBT, a talking therapy during individual and group sessions, also proved highly beneficial. It provided a handy strategy for detecting faulty beliefs and generating healthy, alternative perspectives. The process involved asking ourselves questions like, "Is there any evidence to support my belief?" Followed by, "Is there a different way to look at the situation?" Once we found a new way to see a situation, we set goals to test whether the new belief was valid and helpful. Although I didn't engage with CBT at first, once I found spiritual truths to work with, it helped shift my "stuck" thoughts and supported both holistic and sustainable recovery.

Nutritional Support

Dietetic appointments, as an outpatient and inpatient, were also valuable. The dietitian provided education on nutrition and support with eating. We created meal plans, set weight goals and discussed other queries and concerns. Most treatment facilities also offered dietetic groups, which I looked forward to. These groups provided accurate and up-to-date nutritional information, helping to challenge myths and misconceptions surrounding food. Through them, we also learnt how malnourishment affects the body and the specific intake requirements for regaining and maintaining health. We participated in group activities as well, and questions were always welcomed.

Notably, dietitian appointments were also available after weight restoration, creating a sense of safety and support during the initial stages of recovery and beyond.

Dialectical Behavioural Therapy (DBT)

Another type of talking therapy, DBT, was also offered during individual and group sessions. It provided a way to help regulate emotions and drew on the concept that opposites, like acceptance and change, can work hand in hand. Wise mind statements, mindfulness, self-care and radical acceptance were some skills taught to help manage intense emotions while enabling us to feel present and to move forward. DBT (or the "hippy" version of CBT, as I called it!) was a refreshing, holistic and affirming therapy. It didn't require problem-solving to venture forward and imparted lifelong skills to connect with self, the environment and even God.

Meal Support

Good meal support also played a central role in treatment. It involved well-trained nurses dining with us during inpatient and day programs and helped contain the eating disorder while allowing room for making progress. The nurses role-modelled normal eating, instigated positive talk, knew the dining rules well and had a good understanding of anorexia. Those who were also kind, firm and consistent created a supportive atmosphere and made mealtimes less stressful.

Having meals prepared in the open planned kitchen during the day program aided in normalising mealtimes through seeing, hearing and smelling the preparation process. I also found being served high-quality meals prepared by a cook who followed specific dietetic instructions helped promote health, a sense of worthiness and lowered anxiety at mealtimes too.

Weight Restoration

Weigh-ins were a regular feature of treatment. Although daunting, with holistic support, I found it helpful being expected to gain half to one kilo each week until a BMI of 20. At the day program, once we achieved a BMI of 20, they encouraged us to keep following the dietetic guidelines and to allow our weight to settle at its natural set point, usually between a BMI of 20 and 25. They explained that keeping weight under its set point, even a little, would mean restricting intake/over-exercising, which is unhelpful and may lead to relapse. As people regularly stayed on at the program to help maintain their weight, we also saw what they looked like once recovered. And it was encouraging to see they looked attractive, even vibrant and sounded more optimistic about life.

Exercise Classes

Some treatment facilities also offered exercise/physio classes, which I found beneficial for my body and soul. They ran three times a week, for thirty minutes in the gym, under the guidance of a trained instructor. The classes included stretches, weights, and cardio exercises, and were tailored to individual treatment plans. They helped build strength and fitness levels as weight increased and assisted energy levels and digestion. The instructor also explained what healthy exercise involves and the value of rest. As a result, this helped to decrease anxiety and build the ability to engage in healthful and enjoyable physical activity—rather than excessive, secretive and compulsive exercise.

Art Therapy

Every facility offered art therapy, providing a healthy outlet for processing and expressing thoughts and feelings. Sometimes, we selected what art or craft activity we'd like to do, such as painting, clay modelling or sewing. Other times, the occupational therapist or nurse would present a creative idea to work with. For example, one time, we were encouraged to cut out magazine images to create a picture of what life is like with an eating disorder and what life may look like without one. My life with anorexia was depicted by erupting volcanos and desert lands. For life without anorexia, I cut out a bird flying free and sunlight falling on waterfalls.

N.B. For a more comprehensive look at treatment, please check out the *Resource* section at the back of this book and talk to your local health provider about the treatment options available in your area.

Simple Ways to Support Spirituality

People with anorexia, like anyone, might be on a life-changing spiritual journey of sensing and searching out something beyond themselves and the world we see. For some, like me, it will enable them to find hope and the possibility of recovery when all else fails. A lady in a research article shared, "Without God's help, I would still be extremely sick with no motivation to recover."[20]

I believe this makes it essential to recognise and respect the role spirituality can play in recovery *and* to provide support to explore the spiritual path. Studies also show that thoughts around eating and body image can significantly improve with enhanced spiritual wellbeing.[21] And, "When used appropriately, religion and spirituality in connection with eating disorder treatment and recovery can have a profound effect." Incorporating spirituality in treatment was even shown to give people a sense of purpose and to help them discover meaning in life. It also promoted feelings of self-worth and forgiveness.[22]

So, for health professionals aiming to provide truly effective holistic support, these four suggestions are for you!

1. Consider contacting a chaplain, spiritual director or pastor to discuss spiritual truths and approaches that may help your patient who has a faith. In doing so, you can more readily assist them in discerning lies that feed the disorder and be able to replace them with spiritual truths and practises that bring freedom. You could also collaborate with faith leaders to educate them on anorexia and the support options available, helping to provide holistic care within the community too.

2. Even if your patient doesn't identify with any set ideas about God, this doesn't mean they are void of the possibility of embarking on a life-changing spiritual journey. Because of this, I recommend offering an optional spiritual group during day programs and inpatient treatment. The group needn't prescribe to any one belief system but create a space to explore beliefs, ask questions, reflect, share spiritual experiences and access resources.

3. You could also incorporate spirituality with traditional treatment. Art therapy, DBT, meditation, music therapy, mindfulness, journaling and guided visualisation, for instance, lend themselves to having the ability to support and explore spirituality. You can also easily integrate topics such as hope, peace, love, joy, forgiveness, grace and compassion into traditional therapy models.

4. Lastly, you can support a person's wish to attend chapel, a prayer room or to sit outside in the fresh air so they may have a quiet place to connect with God. They might pray, meditate, sing, journal, read or feel God through nature. Engaging with God looks different for everyone and can occur anywhere. However, a peaceful and private environment

can help promote a sense of sacredness and wellness as the person explores their spirituality.

Caring People

During anorexia, I appreciated and needed every bit of care shown, even if I didn't express it. When people extended care, it displayed beauty and strength, conveyed a message of worthiness, allowed for connection and was never forgotten. Caring people helped usher in life in the face of death.

So, if you are caring for someone with anorexia—I thank you. The heart factor you bring to the journey makes a special difference no amount of treatment alone can achieve. Even if you don't know all the "right things" to say or do, your care and kindness speaks for itself.

At the same time, however, there are certain things you can say and do to help the person along their journey. So, as it's challenging to know what these are, especially as anorexia can make it difficult for people to voice their needs, I am speaking up to offer first-hand advice on what helpful support can look like. As you read, please remember this is a general guide based on my experience; individual needs vary. Nonetheless, I hope it serves you well.

Care-Giving Tips

1. Seek medical advice on behalf of the person if need

2. Listen and allow thoughts and feelings to be voiced

3. Role model healthy eating and positive body image

4. See and relate to them as a person, not a disorder

5. Help practically, for example, offer to drive them to an appointment

6. Remember, anorexia is a complex disorder, and no one is to blame, *including yourself*

7. Cultivate understanding, empathy and wisdom

8. If the person is not up to talking, send a text, email or gift to show you care

9. Consider praying for them in person or alone

10. Show unconditional love, but take care of yourself too!

Reaching Out

If you notice someone is eating less, being preoccupied with food, withdrawing, wearing layers of clothes, over exercising and losing weight, these are signs they may have or develop anorexia. So, as eating disorders are serious, it's important to reach out. Choose a non-mealtime to talk. Be calm, non-judgmental and honest. Try using "I" statements like:

"I am concerned about your health. You look drained and distant," or "I care about you. Is everything okay?" Or "I noticed you are struggling with your eating. How can I support you?"

The next step is to encourage the person to see a doctor who can monitor their health and help them access support services. The sooner they seek help, the better. And people with anorexia need help, no matter how "sick" or not they appear.

Specifically For Parents

Supporting your loved one to access and engage in effective treatment can play a vital role in their path towards health. At the same time, finding reasons to eat, gain weight and recover forms a part of your child's own life journey and takes time. So, although you may desperately want instant health and happiness to appear or to fight the battle on their behalf—patience and understanding are needed the most. Being patient and understanding helps your child feel safe and supported. It also cultivates a sense of hope and love. Even when it feels like you aren't making a difference, you are. Just like a lighthouse keeps shining in the dark, helping boats to navigate their way to the shore, so does your patience, understanding, hope and love.

"I felt devastated and powerless as I watched my daughter succumb to anorexia. Often, they told me that Cassie appeared stuck and treatment-resistant. Nevertheless, as the years passed, I never gave up hope or stopped showing love. Sometimes, it was all I could do. From this, I learnt that both hope and love are essential. We may feel hopeless or like love isn't enough, but through keeping hope alive and continuing to show love, we are doing our best to support the person."

My mum.

Food

Unless you are a health professional or directed otherwise (for instance, parents working with the family-based treatment model), I suggest not commenting on food choices or eating habits during mealtimes—it's a complex matter and saying something that sounds helpful may not be. For instance, it's unhelpful to hear phrases such as, "You're eating well," "Just try a little of this," or "Please eat it for our sake." This is because people with anorexia often feel constrained by many rules about what they can allow themselves to eat and feel unable to break these rules on the spot. They may also be secretly desperate to eat more, so if you praise them for the little they do eat, they may find no reason to increase their intake and may even feel compelled to decrease it. They may also feel guilty, angry, anxious and hateful towards themselves. Instead, try simply serving the food advised by the dietitian, role model normal eating and be available to talk after mealtimes as well.

Communication

Almost always, people with anorexia are portrayed as standing in front of a mirror and perceiving themselves as fat despite being underweight. I never did, and I know of others who say the same. Sometimes I felt fat when I put on weight, but I never thought I looked fat during anorexia. However, being trapped in the disorder, I couldn't always voice what I really thought. If someone asked me, "Do you think you look fat?" I might have even felt compelled to say "Yes." There were times, however, when I felt able to voice my own thoughts, but because I also voiced eating disorder thoughts, people often dismissed what I said. So, as communication can be challenging between the person with anorexia and yourself, my advice is:

- Listen carefully

- Use discernment

- Clarify your understanding

And, above all, show empathy and respect. It's crucial not to judge or deter the person with anorexia from voicing their feelings and thoughts, especially when they're fighting a fierce inner battle to express themselves in the first place.

Specifically For Health Professionals

People with anorexia rely on you for support during their time of darkness and vulnerability. So, I want to encourage you that your words and actions can greatly impact their wellbeing and recovery. For instance, one woman shared that having health professionals believe recovery was possible made her realise:

"Wow, these people have faith in me. I need to have faith in myself."[23]

Not to forget, by showing empathy, consistency and firmness, coupled with having a thorough understanding of anorexia, you can help the person feel safe and supported rather than distressed and drained. By seeing the person behind the disorder and providing holistic and tailor-made treatment, you can also affirm the individual and provide more effective support. Your care makes a world of difference.

Weight

What is the best thing to say to someone about their weight? Nothing. Avoid commenting on weight directly and indirectly, even if it sounds positive and helpful to you, for to them, it very well may not. For instance, refrain from saying: "You're looking better now you've put on weight," or "You don't look so thin now," or even, "You're looking much healthier." These remarks can make the person feel very self-conscious, trigger highly negative thoughts and make them second guess whether they should eat and if they look fat or will look fat once fully recovered. Similarly, if you are concerned about someone's weight loss, instead of focusing on the outside and saying, "Gee, you've lost weight," at an appropriate time, try asking, "Is everything okay?" This is especially important in the initial stages of anorexia when affirming weight loss can unintentionally encourage harmful dieting.

In fact, unless you are a health professional, I suggest to avoid commenting on people's weight altogether. There are far more notable aspects of a person. You can make a positive impact by speaking truths such as, "I enjoy being with you," or "You're beautiful, inside out," or "You're an intelligent and caring person."

Be mindful about commenting on your own weight, too, whether negative or not, because it can inadvertently reinforce the lie that weight is such a significant aspect of who we are—when we know that's not true.

Specifically For Friends

If you have a friend with anorexia, my best advice is to relate to them just like you always have. You aren't a therapist, so there's no pressure to say all the "right words," just be yourself. It is wise, however, not to talk about food and weight, but you don't have to avoid the fact that your friend has an eating disorder. You can ask them, "How can I help?" And express your concern. Just don't forget to talk about everyday things too. It helps the person stay connected with life outside of the disorder; it's also healthy for your friendship.

For example, my friend Tanya often wrote to me while I was in treatment, asking how I was and sharing about her everyday life. Tanya's letters made me smile with her familiar sense of humour and how she saw and expressed things. One letter reads:

"Hi. How are you? I'm pretty dandy. How are your friends in hospital? Say hi to them for me. Have you been doing anything interesting lately? Guess where I went last night? Yep, to a concert, how did you guess? Elton John and Billy Joel are the best. They're mad at the piano! I was watching their fingers and was like, 'Wow.' Well, talk soon. Love your best friend, Tanya."

Spiritual

You can support someone spiritually in many ways. For example, you could pray, share your own story of hope, go on nature walks together or read and share (if appropriate) *Spiritual Keys* at the back of this book. Be mindful, however, not to push your beliefs onto the person or offer spiritual advice that may be irrelevant or harmful. For instance, I had scripture passages taken out of context and quoted to me several times, which was unhelpful. You could even see a skilled faith-based counsellor for guidance on what to say. Most of all, I wholeheartedly encourage you to keep seeking hope, peace, love and joy. Likewise, keep pursuing truth and wisdom. In doing so, you'll shine and be able to offer a unique kind of support that guards and uplifts the soul.

Finding Self and a New Reality

People would say, "We want the old Cassie back." *No way*, I'd think to myself. *I'm not going back to my old self and life. That's what I'm getting away from.* So, I felt stuck and unmotivated to step into recovery, unsure of who I would be and what life would hold without anorexia.

I even found a research article where others with lived experience of an eating disorder voiced their concern about being expected to return to their pre-anorexia selves.[24]

Identity proved such a significant topic that the day program had a group dedicated to it. Together, we brainstormed ideas around the question, "Who would I be without the disorder?" We expressed ourselves through art, contemplated our likes and dislikes, discussed our family tree and shared what we learnt through the disorder and how it has shaped us. Staff also encouraged us to reconnect with life outside of treatment to help form a sense of self.

Alongside exploring identity, we discussed what life might look like beyond recovery. For many, the eating disorder interrupts education, career pathways, cultivation of life skills and relationships. So, we had skills to build and futures to envision. Taking bold steps into the unknown can also feel scary, so we unpacked fears around life after anorexia too.

As a result, I started forming some ideas about my identity. I reconnected with parts of myself that I didn't hate, like my love for animals. I gained new life skills and began to re-integrate into society as an adult. So, recovery didn't take me back to my old self and life, as I had feared.

Still, my sense of worth was shaky, self-hate lingered and life without anorexia seemed overwhelming and unappealing.

Little by little, as I walked the spiritual path, however, I started seeing myself and the world around me in a new light. I also began finding answers to deep questions that went unaddressed in treatment, such as, "Who am I?" and "What is my purpose?" It felt like another layer of life opened before my eyes, and exploring this proved more appealing than staying in anorexia.

So, I'd like to highlight three revelations that helped me to see myself and life in a fresh new light, inspiring me to step beyond anorexia. Although personal, they show how spirituality can continue to support holistic recovery. They may even impart hope and change the landscape of your reality too.

Revelation One

In my early twenties, I felt alive in my heart but trapped in my mind. Countless rules and orders governed my thoughts and affected every part of my life. For instance, I had to study for two hours morning and night, eat at even times, take out the rubbish and iron clothes before lunch and dinner. I had to walk up an even number of stairs at the shopping centre and train station. Before bed, I also had to select what clothes to wear for the next two days in colour orders and create goals, which were also in complex number orders.

I set goals to undo all these rules and orders, but it seemed endless, especially since rules and orders dictated my goals. Until "choice" popped into my mind. I didn't fully understand what it meant, but I knew it had a spiritual component, for it unlocked something in my innermost being, and a word alone could not have done that. Afterwards, I noticed when I felt trapped and compelled to obey rules and orders that I indeed had a choice. I could go along with the familiar and "safe" ways of the disorder, or I could choose not to. And, in small ways, I began choosing how to respond in the moment.

Only later did I realise the full significance of this word—*Choice was impacting my life because its meaning was real. I did have a choice. Nothing could entrap or enslave me. Jesus already set me free through his life, death and resurrection.* The words in Galatians 5:1, "It is for freedom that Christ has set us free," were no longer just words from the Bible. Suddenly, I realised this was already my reality. I could step out from my black-and-white world of rules and orders and straight into a reality full of colour and freedom.

Already Free

Realising I was already free and didn't have to step into the unknown was a game changer. I found change exceedingly difficult with starvation and fear, so employing choice, which ushered in a reality that already was, made experiencing freedom much easier. Did it feel scary? Yes, but a good scary, like an exciting roller-coaster ride, because I knew God was with me and I could trust him.

Activating the truth that I had always been free and always had choice, as Jesus had already set me free, further meant that his life, death and resurrection went from being a concept to being as real as the trees, people, thoughts and feelings in and around me. With this, I saw the world in a different light; it was like seeing through a spiritual lens. The world as I had known it quietly dropped into the background, and a new reality full of wonder emerged. Without a doubt, I had come across a far better dimension to life than I had ever known before.

Revelation Two

During recovery, I realised I could fully recover or remain partially recovered. Partial recovery was appealing. It allowed me to hold onto parts of the disorder that worked for me while also exploring life. Having endured much torment through anorexia, arriving at a place of semi-wellness felt relieving, even deceptively good. Yet, I knew partial recovery put me at risk of relapse and that there was more to life than my eating disorder. So, I kept looking for reasons to let anorexia go.

Then, contemplating the path before me, I had another revelation—*I'm not just in a battle against anorexia. It's deeper. I'm in a spiritual battle.* Satan (which means adversary) cannot be, nor overcome, the God of light. Therefore, he seeks to rule and ruin humanity since God loves us, and we reflect the very image of him. With this insight, it now mattered that each lie I believed and agreed with not only strengthened anorexia and weakened who I was but also allowed darkness a foothold in my life.

Having seen much brokenness and despair during my years spent in the psychiatric unit, I couldn't remain indifferent to the works of darkness in or around me. Finally, I had a powerful reason to say "no" to anorexia, even if it meant full recovery.

Made With Purpose

No longer silenced, and armed with a newfound motive to press on, I felt a strong sense of clarity, direction and determination. It felt like my inner warrior had awakened. Though still not keen on the prospect of full recovery, I was now ready to accept it as the outcome of choosing light.

The more I felt alive, the more I identified with my heart's resolution for justice, mercy and equality, just as I had during childhood. By saying "no" to anorexia, I could now more easily focus on the path of purpose that lay before me, which captured and honoured my heart's passion to stand up and help others.

Equipped with a brand new boldness, passion and purpose, I became involved in an outreach ministry, kept setting recovery goals and engaged with treatment that would see me fully recover.

Revelation Three

Approaching full recovery, I began exploring the topic of identity. At the same time, I became aware of how lies had distorted, hidden and attempted to destroy aspects of who I am. With a growing hunger to see things as they are and a need to feel confident and affirmed, I started seeking deeper truths surrounding my identity. Through searching and contemplating, I found:

I am light to the world (Matthew 5:14)
I cannot be condemned (Romans 8:1)
Power, love and self-discipline are mine (2 Timothy 1:7)
I am a child of royalty; I am not a slave (Romans 8:15)
I am rejoiced over (Zephaniah 3:17)

I am chosen and loved (Ephesians 1:4)

I am a work of art, designed with purpose (Ephesians 2:10)

I am free and forgiven (Colossians 1:13)

I am one with God (1 Corinthians 6:17)

My destiny is to rule and reign with God (Daniel 7:27)

As I meditated on these spiritual truths, I discovered new dimensions to my identity that I had never known, and I felt a new level of hope arise. Inspired, I continue to explore identity and read John and Stasi Eldredge's book *Captivating*. Their book helped me to see that being a woman also added significance to my identity. I learnt women have a unique beauty and play a sacred and essential role in helping humankind, co-ruling and reigning on the earth and birthing and/or nurturing life (Genesis 2:18 and 1:28).

Sitting by the lake, pondering identity again, another revelation unfolded—*Beauty is innate and shines from the inside out*. Women often find themselves drawn to things of beauty like precious stones, vibrant colours and designs, flowers and candle-lit dinners. Why? Beauty knows and identifies with beauty.

No sooner had I realised this than another revelation followed—*Beauty creates beauty*. Seashells, songbirds, serene sunsets and rugged mountains all proclaim beauty. When an artist creates, it reflects something of their soul, their very being. We know creation is beautiful, so we know its creator is too. I then remembered, "God created human beings in his image. In the image of God, he created them; male and female, he created them." (Genesis 1:27 NLT). Suddenly, it all came together—*The creator of all things beautiful, who is also beautiful himself, created women, including myself, intrinsically beautiful.*

Undeniable Worth and Intrinsic Beauty

Discovering foundational truths about my identity was like being lifted out of murky waters—only to find myself as white as a lotus flower. As I knew God was real, he loved me and his thoughts were immeasurably above mine; I could trust all he had to say through the scriptures on identity and found peace. I was no longer tossed back and forth with an uncertainty of who I am and my worth, for what God says is true—regardless of my flaws, failings or what others may say. This revolutionised my entire outlook.

I learnt even the intricate details of identity, like personality, gifting, temperament, appearance, likes and dislikes, are valuable to God. Just as sunset skies were created to display their own exquisite set of colours, I came to see, so are we.

Intrigued and uplifted, I stepped beyond anorexia and into sustainable recovery, not lost in condemnation but captivated by the notion that we are indescribably significant and have an intrinsic beauty independent of worldly standards. I also felt empowered, knowing that although I may not always feel loved, worthy and beautiful, I had affirming truths to hold onto, which proclaim I am.

N.B. Being female, my revelation, in part, pertains to women, but it is important to stress that anorexia is not a gender-specific disorder. Eating disorders are also common amongst men, with at least 30% of people with anorexia estimated to be male.[25]

12. Beyond Anorexia

"I doubt Cassie will ever fully recover," confessed one health professional to another. Yet, I did. I had anorexia for ten years and have been free of it for over a decade. I have faced difficult circumstances—but not once have I slipped back into the trap of an eating disorder.

This does not mean I am successful at recovery. I don't believe success or failure comes into the equation. Neither does it mean that my life, head or heart are all sorted, for there are still areas unrelated to anorexia that are certainly a work in progress and will continue to be so. Not to mention recovery was a long journey, which didn't come in a neat box, and I had considerable help along the way.

It does mean, however, that I can voice the truth: "No one is beyond help, and every little step forward counts." Furthermore, I can share what sustainable recovery looks like for the body, soul and spirit. In doing so, I can disperse fears surrounding recovery and offer real encouragement too.

And even while the journey forward may involve relapses for some, I believe these are merely opportunities for deep healing and growth, and complete recovery can still be found.

So, whether you have an eating disorder or are supporting someone who does, I hope this final chapter of *Beautiful Light* inspires you that profound change is possible and the road ahead can be bright.

Brighter Than Before

Sunflowers are renowned for their radiance and resilience, but they need full sun to thrive. Without it, they don't readily bloom. Sunflowers even follow the sun during the day, and in the dark of the night, they turn around so they are well-positioned to meet the sun each new day.

Encountering the God of hope, peace, love and joy and finding truths about who he is and who I am was like entering a sunny new day. With God, my soul found what it needed to cultivate and sustain recovery. People's skills and caring support nurtured and promoted life. As a result, the turmoil, striving, self-criticism and deception that competed with my soul no longer finds fertile ground to take root. Instead, fresh green shoots can sprout up and are free to flourish in their place.

So, I want to share snippets of my life beyond anorexia to encourage you that by finding what the soul needs, along with a good amount of nurture, life, although it's not easy, can look *brighter than before*.

Colour

I should have felt excited, travelling with Youth With A Mission through the outback in an old retro bus to the Kimberleys, but I didn't. I felt flat. It wasn't the same feeling of utter hopelessness I used to have, for peace from God had uprooted major depression and sowed real hope. Yet, staring out the bus window, I certainly felt deflated. I popped on headphones and turned up *Rain* by Creed to full volume. Once at our destination, I jogged through the bushlands. I also talked with friends and prayed. By the following day, something within had shifted, and my joy returned. So, even though I still get down at times, I now know that with self-care, praying and talking to people—light seeps in—depression lifts and all the colours of life return.

Grace

Alone in my granny flat, with my head in my hands, crying my heart out, I asked God for help and forgiveness. I had messed up big time. Once the tears slowed down, I reached for my journal. I etched a cross with leaves and buds emerging. It felt like God was showing me how he saw the situation, that instead of seeing my sin, he saw grace and new life. I then realised, *Hating myself makes little sense because my reality is one of grace.* With self-hate finding no place in my soul, the truth that I am forgiven, cleansed, loved and worthy sank in deeper. The heaviness in my heart left, and like the picture, life looked hopeful once again.

Comfort

Recently, while walking along the beach, a white poodle pounced by. It reminded me of Casper, my stepdad's dog. A sadness that's hard to describe welled up inside. Feeling the coolness of the ocean waves splash at my legs, distracted, I kept walking along the sand, bathing in the sunshine. Driving home, I wept aloud to God, "I miss my stepdad," and, "Tell him I love him." Knowing that the God I talk to also speaks with my stepdad in heaven brought comfort to my soul. Believing that I will see him and others I have lost again someday further brings hope. By practising mindfulness and turning to God during times of loss, I no longer shut down or bottle up sadness—instead, I feel nurtured and uplifted amongst the pain.

Boldness

Sitting at a restaurant the other day, I was considering what to order when my friend decided she knew what I would like and began ordering on my behalf. "No, I won't like that," I boldly interjected. She looked taken aback but then allowed me to choose. *Wow, that was assertive,* I thought to myself. *I'm unsure whether to feel impressed or concerned if I offended her.* Well, the friendship survived, and all those assertive lessons during treatment, which I thought were trivial, worked. Plus, a lot of inner restoration had taken place over the years, enabling me to speak up and not become oppressed. While not my first time being assertive since recovery, it was the most direct I had been, and I must say, it felt good.

Acceptance

Enjoying strawberries and chocolate at a picnic with people I barely knew, I looked downward and noticed my shirt was inside out. I found it amusing, laughed and walked to the bathroom to re-adjust it.

It didn't bother me in the slightest that I may have looked odd with my wardrobe mishap. Yet, it has taken many years for me to feel okay with imperfections. During recovery, my psychologist said, "You did your best in the given circumstance." Her wise words helped me to see things differently and to be kinder to myself. They also fitted with the larger framework I was finding for life—that we were created perfect, in a perfect world, by a perfect God, yet now live in the process of being restored to perfection. This framework further validated my inclination towards perfectionism while helping me accept the tension of the renewal process that our broken world, including myself, are living in. And, as I learnt at the picnic that day, holding onto the tension that imperfection and messiness are okay allows room for unexpected joy and peace to pop up too.

Freedom to Grow

"I can't stand it; that's disgusting. Can you get your pants off the bench?" I snapped at my husband the other night. He had left dirty pants on our breakfast bar again. On reflection, I know I could have managed it differently.

Treatment has taught me how to be assertive in communicating needs. Journalling, sitting with my emotions, going for walks, praying and deep breathing were other skills I also gathered through recovery to help navigate emotions. The spiritual path further showed me that in choosing love, anger dissipates, and peace can arise. And therapy enabled me to see anger is simply a feeling; it doesn't make me a "bad" person, nor do I need to be punished for it or hang my head in shame.

So, on the upside, although my response to the dirty pants incident was not ideal—free from self-criticism and feelings of condemnation—I could reflect on the situation, apologise, learn and not beat myself up in the process.

I must add there have been many times since recovery I have chosen love over anger, even if it has meant retreating to the bathroom, pleading, "God, please help. I'm about to explode!" So, while growth is ongoing, fresh shoots of love towards myself and others have emerged.

Self-Worth

A while ago, entering the nurse's station, I spotted a table set with afternoon tea. It was my last day of nursing at the little country hospital, and the staff had thrown a farewell party—just for me. I felt honoured, surprised and loved. Yet, I hadn't always felt so accepted or even liked. For quite some time, I felt like the odd one out. I was the new girl from the city with barely any work experience. A few nurses gave me a hard time, and I felt awkward sitting in the dining room on meal breaks. Naturally,

I wanted them to like and include me, yet having found my own values, self-worth and identity during recovery—I no longer *needed* people to like or include me. Using DBT and CBT skills also helped with challenging feelings and automatic assumptions. And in the end, although not everyone liked me, that didn't matter. I formed many wonderful friendships, thoroughly enjoyed nursing and left feeling blessed.

Present Living

I had intended, for a long time, to go on another mission trip. Then, last year, praying by the bay, I felt God say, "Go on a holiday with Aaron instead. Explore, laugh, connect and invest in each other. Immerse yourself in my love and glory for now. Missions can wait. Focus on me, my love and restoration."

How ironic—God was saying not to serve others but to go on a holiday instead. Clearly, he is not the rule-based God I thought him to be growing up.

In fact, during recovery, I learnt it was religious people Jesus corrected while on earth for being rule-orientated instead of love centred. So, although I feel free from having to keep rules or standards to be a "good" Christian, I can still slip into striving and forget to live in the moment, laugh and love. But that's okay. God reminds me, as he did by the bay, that the spiritual life is not one of "good works," fulfilling expectations or unhealthy striving. Instead, it's about living in the present moment with him, where all goodness flows.

New Delights

Oh, how I miss my childhood home dearly! Yet, I now have my own home, and Aaron and I have a beautiful little daughter. So, not only have my surroundings changed since anorexia, but so has my homelife. No longer do my parents' struggles affect me, partly because I have moved away but also because I have come to know God as my father. Knowing he is always available, comforts, provides, encourages, protects and never leaves—brings peace and healing to my soul. It even frees me to enjoy my relationship with my parents to the fullest and to reflect with gratefulness for the loving upbringing that I experienced.

These days, I also have new areas of homelife to explore. I enjoy creating a healthy, peaceful atmosphere in the home. My husband and I love the ocean, so we have an interior coastal theme happening. Hosting kids' parties is fun too! There are also new relationship dynamics to both enjoy and navigate as a mother and wife. So, beyond anorexia, my homelife has evolved, bringing new delights and further growth opportunities too.

Peace Along the Path

A few nights ago, I took out my iPhone, clicked on the notes app and began jotting down my weekly plan and a few goals. Tired, I closed the app before finishing and hopped into bed. And that was that. I may achieve some goals, forget what I wrote, or something unexpected might happen and my plans could completely change.

I'm not exactly sure how I have become so relaxed with plans and goals, but I know I have found peace and freedom in realising it's not all up to me to achieve—God is at work, helping me to learn, grow and be fruitful. With knowing God and who I am, goals no longer define or control me, nor do they have the power to make me feel good, bad or entrapped. Planning and goal setting are simply tools I now use to help me along the path of life. And often, I'm at peace to see them shaped and shifted, knowing the process allows colours to appear and life to break through.

Body, Food & Wellbeing

It's true, at the core, anorexia is not about the body or food. Nonetheless, I did fear recovery would mean losing self-discipline with exercising and eating and that I would look like I did before the disorder and feel awful all over again. I even feared trusting God would make me fat, believing he only cared about my heart, not my body.

However, interwoven through the recovery process, I discovered new ways of self-discipline, eating, exercising, managing feelings and challenging thoughts. I also found wisdom, peace and the ability to love myself, or at least to be kinder to self. And the truth that God is the author of holistic, healthy living emerged. As a result, through drawing on all I had and was discovering—my body and food fears didn't come true. On the other side of anorexia, I found a healthier lifestyle and a higher level of wellbeing than I had ever known.

So, I'm eager to share what I found in place of my body and food fears. I hope this inspires you that through the recovery journey, our body image and how we exercise and eat can also change for the better.

For the Better - Body

Weight

*I feared returning to a healthy weight would equate
to being unhappy and unattractive.*

Today, however, my weight is within the healthy BMI range, which simply means my weight is healthy. Feeling alive within, I'm also more interested in life itself than what I weigh. My self-perception and values have also evolved, affecting how I see myself. I now see being my natural weight doesn't make me unattractive, and my husband certainly agrees. And although I am around the same weight as I was before anorexia, it sits on me differently as a woman, and I like that. To my relief, being an adult also means I can explore a variety of stores and find clothes that suit me instead of being limited to the kid's department, where clothes often didn't fit as a preteen. I can also choose outfits ranging across three sizes without thinking twice about the numbers. I now know that sizing differs from brand to brand, and I don't tie my identity to my size. Even though I occasionally think *I would like to look slimmer*, self-hate no longer arises. Instead, I can adjust my eating if needed or, more often than not, choose to let go of the thought and go about my day.

Appearance

I thought I would hate my appearance all over again once I recovered.

What I found was the opposite. Most days, I now feel at peace with how I look. I like my brunette hair and brown eyes that I once deemed plain and boring. Being short isn't something I think negatively about anymore, either. Actually, my height comes in handy, especially when playing with kids. I have no problem with having acne, even though I'm over thirty years old! My nose is obviously the same size and shape it was when I disliked it, but now, I don't even think about it. I like my olive skin and how it reflects my Aboriginal and Italian heritage. I like that I now have strong calves too. My new outlook reminds me a little of the children's book *I Love Me* by Sally Morgan and Ambelin Kwaymullina (I highly recommend this book).[26] I wouldn't say I love myself, but with time, having my innermost needs met and holding onto truths—I am starting to appreciate parts on the inside and outside of me.

Exercise

I feared that without harsh rules, I would stop exercising altogether.

These days, I no longer adhere to harsh exercise rules, and although I don't exercise as much as I did during anorexia—thank goodness—I still regularly exercise. By learning to listen to wisdom and my body and incorporating what I learnt about physical activity during treatment, I exercise freely for about 40 minutes most days. I think of it as self-discipline, lined with grace and choice. Depending on the weather and how I feel, I walk, jog, go to the gym or aqua aerobics. I also make sure I'm well-hydrated. My fitness level isn't fantastic, but it's better than before anorexia. Recently, I even jogged non-stop around my old school oval for the very first time. I may have looked like *Forest Gump*, but it felt good! I also have muscle tone in areas of my body that I never had before. Notably, I can rest if I am tired, unwell or want a break, and I can re-engage with exercise at any time too.

Socialising

I believed recovery would leave me feeling shy
and self-conscious like before.

To be honest, I did feel self-conscious when I first gained weight, and people commented. However, that period was short-lived. Although sometimes I feel shy, I'm now okay with being an introvert. Most times, however, I'm not shy and am more socially outgoing than prior to anorexia. Even if I feel unsatisfied with how I look, unlike before, I still go out, and once I'm out and about, I forget about my appearance and freely engage with people and enjoy the moment. *Time Tested Beauty Tips* by Sam Levenson, one of Audrey Hepburn's favourite poems, says,

"For beautiful eyes, look for the good in others; for beautiful lips, speak only words of kindness..."[27]

Like the poem, I now see there's an element of beauty that only appears in connection with others, and I carry that truth with me. Along with collecting truths and forming my own values, after being isolated for so long during anorexia, I simply appreciate being in the moment and my social connections more now than ever before.

Confidence

I feared that without anorexia, I would lose self-confidence.

My fear, once again, didn't come true. I now have a newfound confidence. I wear clothes and accessories that I like and which express my personality. My wardrobe comprises silk wrap skirts, bamboo shirts, fair-trade earrings, comfy jeggings, second-hand knit cardigans and old boots. Unlike in my early teens, I now feel free to wear my hair out, messy or tied back for convenience. During the onset of anorexia, although I found the confidence to wear tight jeans and midriff shirts, this confidence depended on my looks and not caring about myself, anyone else or life in general. It was superficial. Today, however, I have a new confidence grounded in truths about who I am. If I forget these truths, music that makes my soul sing, prayer, being in nature or a kind word from a friend—all help me remember who I am and to feel confident again. Not only does this confidence affect how I look and feel, but how I interact too. No longer do I nervously look downwards when I walk. Instead, I look straight ahead and can smile and say, "Hi," when people pass by.

For the Better - Food

Balanced Eating

I feared that after depriving myself for so long, I'd overeat "forbidden" foods once I recovered.

Admittedly, even though I felt drawn to carbs and sweets during early recovery, and I overate them at times, it never spun out of control. I kept aiming to eat three balanced meals and snacks each day. I increasingly tuned into my body, addressed health issues, nourished my soul and gradually developed a desire for healthy eating.

So, now, I eat a healthy diet, which includes a variety of nutritious foods from every food group, being mindful of portion sizes and limiting foods I am intolerant to. For instance, I eat salmon, dark chocolate, bananas, nuts, crackers with hummus, yoghurt, eggs, fresh honey and veggie juices. As healthy eating involves wisdom, freedom and choice, I also eat foods I once considered "forbidden" in smaller quantities (sometimes I still overdo it, and that's fine) and foods that aren't "super" healthy, out of convenience and to fit my budget. I enjoy cakes on special occasions and licking the wooden spoon when making them too!

Before anorexia, I only had a vague idea about healthy eating, and I didn't greatly value it. I also developed extreme ideas. Yet, with treatment, exploring holistic health and getting to know the creator of nature and all its goodness—I now prefer and enjoy healthy eating.

Self-Regulation

I feared letting food be food, not a source of help or comfort.

With practising self-care, employing DBT skills and finding spiritual truths, food no longer takes the role of reward or punishment in my life. My emotions have also become something to embrace, not suppress or fear.

Even though I still comfort eat sometimes, like I did before anorexia, it's different. Now, when feeling drawn to food, I can pause, pray if needed, tune into my hunger levels and remind myself that *It's good for my body and soul to sit, relax and eat a well-prepared meal.* I can then choose whether to eat in a healthy manner, tend to my emotions or simply move on from the distraction of food.

Importantly, I am now much kinder to myself. So, if I comfort eat, I don't beat myself up about it. Life is not perfect, and neither am I, and that's okay. I have even discovered that consuming a few extra chocolates doesn't affect my weight. Most of all, I am free to try again (and again) to let go of unhelpful coping mechanisms, knowing each moment presents new opportunities for self-discovery and growth.

Enjoyment

I feared enjoying food would result in a loss of self-discipline.

Contrary to what I feared, I found enjoyment and self-discipline can co-exist! Mindfully enjoying food can even help me feel present and more able to exercise self-discipline.

So, these days, I enjoy food, whether alone or with others. As food no longer dominates or clouds social gatherings, I can also enjoy the company, aromas, music and ambience that often go hand in hand with eating and being social.

My world of dining out has further evolved, being older on the other side of anorexia. These days, I look forward to trying trendy new restaurants, catching up with friends over a cappuccino, hosting guests and having the rare alcoholic drink. I also enjoy eating without comparing my food or serving size to others, which feels liberating.

Occasionally, when I feel hesitant to enjoy food, I "just do it" or recall the words of Jesus, "The thief comes only to steal, kill and destroy; I have come that they may have life, and have it to the full" (John 10:10). In doing so, I find the courage and freedom to keep enjoying.

Hunger and Satiety

I feared being in the moment and listening to my appetite.

Listening and responding to my appetite has been a journey but nothing to fear. Although I felt like both an empty pit and overly full at times during recovery, after reaching and sustaining my natural weight, my hunger and satiety levels balanced out. I also discovered that through mindfulness and continuing to eat well, my body has a "stop point" when eating, so I can listen to it and trust it. As a result, I can get seconds if I'm hungry or leave some food on my plate. I can eat flexibly and refrain from painfully measuring all my food. I can also "sit" with uncomfortable feelings, listen to wisdom and recall truths that set me free. So, if feeling empty reminds me of starvation, I remind myself that *The feeling is temporary; I can grab something to eat.* If I am exceptionally full, I know that *The feeling will pass, my weight will likely remain unchanged and who I am isn't connected to how much I've eaten.*

Most of the time, however, hunger and satiety are just a part of everyday life. Through recovery, I have gained trust in the design of my body and a new level of peace and self-mastery.

Speaking Up

I feared saying "Yes" and "No" to food.

As a kid, I often said, "Yes, thank you," to food to please people. During anorexia, I declined food to appease the disorder. Then, entering recovery, I feared others would interpret my "No, thank you" to food as the "eating disorder voice" rather than my own. Or if I said, "Yes, please," people would assume I was completely better.

Now, none of this is an issue. Over time, by employing assertive skills and holding onto my values, I have learnt to speak up and care for myself regarding food choices. Today, I can say, "No, thank you," or "Yes, just a little," or simply, "Yes, please."

Having the freedom to accept or decline food feels empowering. For instance, one night after dinner, I visited a family who were poor. Unknowingly, the wife had spent all day preparing a large meal. I wasn't hungry but said nothing and accepted her food with thanks. I wasn't doing this out of fear or obligation, but because it aligned with my values. My gosh! I was exceedingly full that night, but it was a once-off event, and I was honestly glad to have said, "Yes, please."

Words of Life

During the height of anorexia, I compulsively journaled multiple times a day. Angry, exaggerated and swear words about my eating and weight filled the pages. My handwriting was tiny and extremely neat or irregular, messy and straying off the lines. Then, one day, reaching for my journal, I realised, *I'm journalling as if I'm answerable to someone, reporting to them through my negative writing*. It felt dark and controlling. I stopped journaling that same day.

Not long after, I heard other people with anorexia share about the "eating disorder voice." It was a voice within their mind that went beyond self-criticism. The voice was condemning, controlling, tormenting, spoke lies and instilled fear. It reminded me of how I felt under the control of something separate from myself when giving accounts in my journal.

After realising how this "voice" affected both myself and others, I continued challenging and rejecting eating disorder thoughts while renewing my mind with truths. And as I journeyed forward, I began finding the freedom to express my heart. At first, my journal only contained a few words that conveyed what I really believed, accompanied by eating disorder thoughts. Yet, with time, I grew stronger and more skilled at discerning and expressing myself without the "eating disorder voice" tagging along. Then, at nineteen years old, I jotted down what I was thankful for each day:

September 2000

"I'm thankful for the gorgeous weather, healthier hair and nails, inner peace and my kind bus driver."

Three years later, they asked me to write a weekly self-evaluation report during the day program. Feeling safe and supported, knowing that my nurse would read it, I continued to express thoughts and feelings outside of the eating disorder. So, at twenty-two years old, I wrote:

November 2003

"I have been feeling unwell, tired and down at times. However, I met with some church friends at *Gloria Jean's* on Friday night. I enjoyed talking with them. I also enjoyed seeing Tanya's band at the *Roxy* Theatre. I have eaten better as well, but still feel stuck in some areas. I'm looking forward to seeing my sister next week."

Step by step, my journal entries changed, reflecting true feelings, inner life and freedom. These days, I freely write when I want to. I express an array of emotions and thoughts and often draw pictures. I also like "mind mapping," where I choose a topic and creatively write words that resonate with my soul around it. I find it therapeutic. For instance, if I select the topic of *Self-Care*, I might write in shades of green around *Self-Care*:

"Sipping peppermint tea, deep breathing
and rest—nourishment for the soul."

What I enjoy most, however, is hearing from God and recording what he says. I've learnt God doesn't usually (although sometimes does) speak in an audible voice. Rather, he is spirit and communicates via our spirit in a quiet, gentle, loving, affirming and life-giving way. Hearing from him is like walking along the beach, unaware of the continuous splashing sound of the waves until we tune into them. So, now, I regularly ask God, "What do you want to say to me?" And I write what I sense impressed on my heart. Sometimes, I don't hear well; the world and my head can be noisy, but other times, I hear him so clearly. Let me share some of these journal entries too:

April 2012

"Rich in colour as a rainbow, knitted together, I formed you. I delight in you; gems and riches are your story. Elegance and captivated beauty is how I see you. Stand and be counted, do not shy, do not fret, be bold and be strong, for I, your God, am with you to the end. I long for engagement, true engagement, candles and a meal shared. Countless worth are my people. Colours poured onto butterfly wings—so I have designed you and designed you well. You're my beloved, precious child, woman of God."

May 2013

"You are like a wildflower at times, hungry and free. You are like a sunflower at times, bathing in me. You are like a golden sunset on the sea to me, and you arise after dark times and keep on shining. You try to run and hide. I seek you out, and I carry you. You need not to fear. My armour is on you. You are not alone. Can you sense I am near? We can tread on new ground and in new ways. Nothing is impossible with me. I need your entire heart, dear child. Your life ahead is good. I have planned it and ordained it from day one. Though you stumble and fall, I am always near. I redeem all your ways. The cross shines through your life. Your life and mine are one. That's how close I am. That's how much I love and adore you. I sing over you. I will always sing over you. Break forth into this new season. Bells are ringing. It's your wedding day. Brides are walking, tall and strong."

(Unknowingly, at the time, three of my friends and
I would all soon become brides.)

Why Share This?

It feels good to be free. I am no longer enslaved, tormented or silenced. I can freely connect with and express my heart. It's something worth sharing and celebrating!

On top of this, hearing from God and writing what he says has been one of the greatest joys I have discovered beyond anorexia—it is also my lifeline. When doubts arise and hard times set in, I hold onto his words of life and truth, and my soul remains restored and free.

For people with anorexia, I hope by sharing how my journal entries, which reflect my soul, have profoundly changed, inspires you to keep pursuing your freedom and to express your heart. And as the harsh and controlling voice within the disorder can feel relentless, I also hope you feel encouraged that there is a life-giving voice to tune into instead.

So, it seems fitting that I should end by asking, "God, what do you want to say to the readers?" I sense him say:

"Begin a journey of hope, and you will find me and all the pieces of life will come together. Be lifted up, for I lift and embrace you and all your needs. Nothing is too much for me. You are not too much for me. I am pleased with you. I spent my life on you. I adore you, and you captivate me. I am always here for you. I am for you and not against you. Come to me, and I will give you true rest. Light piercing through darkness, I am he."

AFTERWORD

While writing *Beautiful Light,* I came across a research paper on eating disorders that found, "Strong and internalised religious beliefs coupled with having a secure and satisfying relationship with God were associated with lower levels of disordered eating, psychopathology and body image concern."[28]

This suggests, what my story highlights, that spirituality can play a significant role in recovery. For me, encountering God brought hope—despite the severity of my disorder. When coupled with effective treatment and caring support, holistic recovery emerged. So, I want nothing more than for *Beautiful Light* to have likewise offered you tangible hope. Hope that no matter how dark it may seem, light can break through and the path forward can appear.

For people with anorexia, I hope my story has brought you peace in knowing you're not alone; that I (and others) can also identify with the darkness the disorder brings and yet can testify that there is light, not at the end of the tunnel, but in reach, where you are at. I also hope sharing my experience of overcoming anorexia and what life can look like beyond the disorder has encouraged and equipped you on your venture forward. Perhaps most of all, I hope *Beautiful Light* has inspired you spiritually and that you find rays of light and truths that set you free. May the words "You are worthy" echo throughout your journey, and your soul find what it longs for.

To those who offer support, I hope you have found a deeper understanding of the disorder and how spirituality can help pave the way forward. I also hope you feel inspired that a holistic approach to treatment is beneficial and that *Beautiful Light* enhances the support you already give. Equally so, my heart longs that you take away the truth that each time you show care and understanding to someone struggling with anorexia, you make a positive difference.

In particular, for health professionals helping someone through the disorder, I thank you. Your skills, knowledge and care bring relief and uphold life. Family and friends—your love does the same. Deep down, I also hope that my story has encouraged you in your personal life, for we all share universal soul needs, and so lays truths and gems in my story that pertain to us all.

Last of all, to every reader, in choosing *Beautiful Light*, a book that speaks of hope and understanding, I believe it reflects something of your heart. Something that is truly good and actively seeks to find light and honour life. That itself is powerful, precious and worth pursuing.

In closing, I want to share these poetic words that resonate with my soul, "Deep cries out to deep" (Psalm 42:7).

Anorexia took me to a place of darkness. Yet, God heard my heart's silent cry, reached deep and delivered me to a place of light—a place of finding, being and experiencing life to the fullest. I can now say, without a doubt:

Life is not easy nor perfect, but it is bright
and full of colour beyond the long night of anorexia.

ACKNOWLEDGEMENTS

People who were loving, patient, understanding and kind for the duration of my disorder kept a flicker of light going in the dark. Then, others came along for short periods but shined at crucial points. So, I want to express my heart-filled gratitude to everyone who helped me along my journey, with a special note of thanks to these bright lights:

Sarah, my psychologist, shined. She was a positive role model, honest, compassionate, bubbly and confident. Sarah also had sound insight into anorexia and how it affected me. I didn't need to explain or justify myself. She listened and showed sincere care and understanding, helping me to feel relieved and supported. She imparted skills that worked for me, such as mindfulness and listening to wisdom—enabling me to feel present, safe and empowered. Importantly, Sarah respected my spiritual beliefs and accredited my faith as playing a significant role in my recovery. She even went the extra mile to support me as I faced new challenges. For instance, after sharing my anxiety about clothes shopping, she said, "Go shopping, and if it gets too overwhelming, take a moment out and text me if you need to." To my benefit, Sarah believed recovery was possible and cheered me on each step of the way.

My dietitian at the adult psychiatric unit was a much-needed ray of light. She understood well the implications of anorexia on the body and soul and had a kind and caring approach. She held our consultations outside in the fresh air, and when I was well enough, we went for walks together, talking along the way. One time, we came across a little chapel. She lit a candle for me, saying, "Cassie, you really must get better. I'm having dreams about you at night!" And though I often voiced fears and frustrations, she patiently listened and responded firmly but fairly. She corrected faulty beliefs about food, but ever so gently, referring to my thoughts as "magical thinking." Unfortunately, my dietitian didn't see the fruit of her hard labour, but she did sow seeds towards recovery and made me feel safe and cared for at my worst.

The clinical director and the staff at the day program also shined. The director was consistent with being caring and firm. He sat next to me one mealtime, a meal I didn't eat. Afterwards, he said, "It must feel horrible. I don't know what you're going through, but you can't not eat your food." He understood how anorexia worked, spoke to me as Cassie—not a disorder—equipped me with CBT skills and ran a program that ultimately saw me recover.

At the day program, Nurse "Tia" also showed care, respect, understanding and patience and went out of her way to help. She even made personalised colourful affirmation cards in her own time for us patients to keep. I still have these. She related to people with eating disorders as ordinary people and shared a little about her own struggles and triumphs. With expertise, care and compassion, they helped me feel supported and nurtured as I recovered.

Mum was like a candle that never went out. She encouraged me to see our doctor when I initially lost weight, liaised with the eating disorder team and was involved in all my treatment. Through notes, words, gifts and actions, Mum conveyed love. She drove daily to visit me in hospital and helped in any way possible with schooling, shopping, washing clothes, etc. Most of all, Mum was ready to listen any time, day or night. I frequently voiced my fears, anxieties and frustrations, yet she didn't try to correct my thoughts or emotions but had empathy and wisdom to share.

When I would cry inconsolably, Mum would say, "This feeling won't last forever." So, right and soothing were her words. At times, I pushed Mum away, as I feared feeling anything at all, especially love. Mum, however, never pushed me away. She walked with me every step of the way, not only through anorexia but life before and after it, too, in unconditional love, forbearance and grace.

Dad came alongside me and kept encouraging me to fight anorexia and to comply with treatment so I had the best chance of recovery. He spoke highly of me as his "intelligent and caring" daughter and didn't let the disorder change his mind. Dad helped practically by visiting me in treatment, advocating for increased government support for eating disorder facilities, spending one-on-one time together and keeping in regular contact with doctors. He also made friends with other patients when visiting me in psychiatric units. It didn't bother Dad that some patients had major mental and behavioural issues. I never told him this positively affected me, but it did; it warmed my heart. Dad hugged me, cried and persevered in love, a special type fathers have.

Kim, my stepdad, affirmed me, delighted in me and involved himself in my world during my childhood and early teens. On the other side of anorexia, he continued to show interest in my life and wellbeing. During the disorder, Kim had moved interstate. Even so, he kept in touch and saw me at pivotal times. He frequently visited when I was first hospitalised for anorexia, when I was seriously ill with pneumonia and for my twenty-first birthday. He talked with Mum to find out how I was doing and sent cards and gifts. Kim was like a candle that flickered and shined at just the right times. He rarely shared what was on his mind but always hugged me before leaving the hospital with tears welling up, saying, "You know I love you, Poss (short for possum) and want to see you better."

My Pastor Paul role-modelled a life inspired by and immersed in God, emanating hope and passion to step beyond the ordinary. He wrote to me in hospital, offered to visit and came to my twenty-first party. Paul prayed for me, always asked how I was and didn't tell me I had to change. He also listened to and heard well from God and preached life-giving words that spoke to my heart. Through his teachings, I learnt I could hear from God too. He welcomed feedback and questions throughout the church service, which helped me to feel present, affirmed and included. He encouraged us to get involved in what God was doing, and at the end of each gathering, we prayed for one another. With this, I learnt about my relationship with God, experienced a caring community and gained much-needed spiritual direction.

My friends sparkled brightly, extending their love and friendship when I had nothing to give in return. We didn't spend a lot of time together during anorexia. Yet my friends consistently sent cards and letters, attended special events like birthday parties, asked Mum how I was doing and offered practical help. My closest friends, *Tanya, Sharon, Fiona and Dianna,* were also there for me once I recovered, lighting up life beyond anorexia with laughter and warmth and supplying a sense of safety in my changing world. Dianna, my friend since kindergarten, wrote a poem for me. Di was only in high school when she wrote it. However, she was brave enough to let me know that she cared about me and that it affected her to see me struggling with anorexia. I valued her poem. I remember these lines by heart:

> "I know how sad you're feeling and how hard life can be,
> This poem is to remind you that you have a friend in me.
> I won't tell you to smile or be brave, but that true
> happiness you alone can pave."

RESOURCES

Eating Disorder Hope

An online community that offers a range
of holistic eating disorder support

www.eatingdisorderhope.com

Butterfly Foundation

Information and support for people with
eating disorders and their carers

www.butterfly.org.au

Jenni Schaefer

Author and motivational speaker with lived
experience of an eating disorder

www.jennischaefer.com

Australian National Eating Disorder Helpline

8 am-midnight (AEST), 7 days a week. 1800 ED HOPE (1800 33 4673)

Recovery Warriors

Support for people with eating disorders, offering tools and guidance

www.recoverywarriors.com

InsideOut Institute

Research and information hub on eating disorders

www.insideoutinstitute.org.au

Destiny Haven

A residential recovery place for women in the Hunter Valley, Australia

www. destinyhaven.org.au

Tastelife

Education and support for people with
eating disorders and their carers

www.tastelifeuk.org

Rock Recovery

Support groups and therapy for people with eating disorders

www.rockrecoveryed.org

SEEKING SUPPORT

There are many paths to recovery, and each person's journey is unique. Since anorexia is a serious and complex disorder, however, that impacts the whole person, individuals often need professional support to stay safe and recover. So, below is a simple (not exhaustive) guide to help you navigate treatment if you're seeking support for yourself or someone you love.

First Step

People often say, "The earlier the intervention, the better."[29] I'd add the earlier *effective intervention* is accessed, the better. So, if you or someone you know is struggling and may have anorexia, I encourage you to see a doctor who has good insight into eating disorders. The doctor may then refer you/your loved one to a treatment service that can offer the best level of support.

Levels of Support

Outpatient Support - Typically comprises a team of doctors, psychologists, dietitians and nurses who work together to support someone with anorexia in their community. It also enables people to maintain contact with family, friends and society while recovering.

Day Programs - These offer supervised meal support and individual and group therapy during the day while patients continue to live in their homes, allowing them to stay connected with their family, friends and day-to-day life.

Residential Care - Provides medical monitoring, meal support and individual and group therapy in a residential setting where people stay overnight but may return home on weekends.

Inpatient Care - This can involve hospitalisation to treat medical complications related to anorexia. It can also help to improve eating and weight or provide people with more intense support if suicidal thoughts are present.[30]

Standard Therapies

Within community settings and eating disorder programs, you will find different kinds of therapies that support mental, emotional and physical health. Some of the main options include:

Individual Therapy - This is where a psychologist helps to explore and manage thoughts, emotions and behaviours in a healthy way that supports recovery. They may use cognitive behavioural therapy (CBT) to help replace unhelpful thoughts with healthy ones. Or other therapies like dialectical behavioural therapy (DBT) to help manage strong emotions through mindfulness, distress tolerance, radical acceptance and emotional regulation.

Medical Treatment - Usually, this involves seeing a doctor who can provide physical assessments, education, referrals and arrangements for hospitalisation if needed. It can also include seeing a psychiatrist who can offer psychological support and prescribe medication if required.

Nutritional Support - This is where a dietitian helps people with anorexia and their families understand the interaction between food, nutrition and wellbeing. The dietitian also provides meal plans and supports achieving and maintaining a healthy weight.

Family-Based Treatment - Entails a therapist guiding the parents to help their child/teen with eating, weight restoration, and managing their own symptoms and wellbeing. It is a popular therapy and aims to help the young person recover at home with the support of their family.[31]

Complementary Therapies

In addition to standard therapies, there's a range of complementary treatments to choose from that support holistic recovery. Many of these are available in the community, and some treatment services offer them too. For instance:

Equine Therapy - This involves interacting with horses to promote healing. For example, it can help to reveal a person's core beliefs through how they respond to the horse. Caring for a horse also requires focus, which encourages being in the moment and presents an opportunity to nurture and feel love in return.

Meditation - Is a practice that aims to decrease stress levels while feeling present and promoting body awareness. It can support relaxation, sleep and digestion too. People can engage in it anywhere, but there are also

24/7 prayer rooms accessible to the public, free of charge across Australia, where people can meditate, reflect and pray.

Faith-based Counselling - This is where traditional therapy techniques combine with spiritual beliefs and practices to bring a deep and richer experience to the recovery journey. It can also include prayer ministry, healing through guided imagery, breath prayers and meditation.

Movement Therapy - Promotes connection with the body, being in the moment, and focusing on what the body can do rather than what it looks like. It also provides an opportunity for self-expression, healthy emotional regulation and the chance to experience positive feelings too.[32]

For further information on seeking support, please check out the online sites listed in this resource section and talk with your local health provider.

SELF-HELP

$\mathcal{B}$esides accessing treatment, there are many things you can do to help create your own path forward. This is why self-help is so good; you can explore and choose what works best for you. So, here are a few ideas to get you started:

1. Experiment With Self-Care

Long showers, buying flowers, applying essential oils, taking naps or going on mindful walks are some of the self-care activities I enjoy. Since we are all different, however, I encourage you to list self-care activities that appeal to you and, one-by-one, give them a go! It may feel hard at first, but with practice, self-care can become a helpful way to deal with distress while instilling a sense of self-worth. It's also a wonderful way to experience nurture and the present moment.

2. Create Tailor Made Resources

Try bookmarking online eating disorder support sites that speak to you. You may also like to add online support groups to your resources, such as those offered through *The Butterfly Foundation* at butterfly.org.au or *Beat Eating Disorders* at www.beateatingdisorders.org.uk. Recovery apps, like Recovery Warrior's *Rise Up + Recover* app, are also handy tools. And don't forget to include inspiring books like *Life Without Ed* by Jenni Schaefer and *Hidden Hunger* by Maxine Vorster.

3. Explore Spiritual Practices

Spiritual practices can help with distressing thoughts and feelings and cultivate a sense of wellbeing. Meditation is a popular choice for people of all faiths. Declaring truths and turning scripture into prayer can also help to renew the mind and uplift the soul. Breath prayers, *Praise Moves* (postures coupled with scriptures) and worship are other practices to explore. I've tried them all and recommend each one.

4. Get Creative

Creativity is a healthy way to express ourselves, bless others and gain a sense of satisfaction, healing and joy. Art, photography, music, dance, writing, woodwork, decorating and designing are some ideas that pop to mind. You can get creative on your own, with your therapist or join a class. What I like best about creativity is that there are no standards to meet or rules to follow—everyone is free to be creative in their own way.

5. Collect "Words of Wisdom"

Grab some coloured paper, a journal or sticky notes and write "words of wisdom" to meditate on. You might make up your own, recall words your therapist or even grannie once said, or find inspiration through the net, books and songs. Here are a few of my favourites:

"Rest is a requirement, not a reward."
"Having a bad day doesn't undo all the progress you've made."
"This feeling won't last forever."

6. Be Pro-Active with Social Media

Follow inspiring media that aligns with your values. I found through following pages featuring flowers that my *Facebook* newsfeed has blooms popping up everywhere, which feels uplifting, especially on hard days. Similarly, follow and like recovery sites too. At the same time, turn off media "likes" and unfollow accounts that are triggering and make you feel inadequate. You can even schedule media holidays and use digital wellbeing apps to help set time limits on your media use. Make media work for you!

7. Discover Your Passions

What makes your heart come alive? Perhaps it's hard to know since anorexia can be all-consuming, but that's okay—it gives you the chance to explore old passions and discover new ones too. For instance, you could volunteer at an animal shelter, pursue photography, support a charity, join an art class, bushwalk or quietly watch the sunrise. Uncovering our passions not only distracts us from distressing feelings but can also bring joy and reveal parts of our identity and purpose too.

8. Design an Action Plan

It might include an eating, self-care and social goal to work on each week. The *Recovery Record* is a helpful little app for this. Remember, however, that goals don't define us, and no one always meets them perfectly. They are simply a tool to help us. You may want to ask for help with your action plan too. A strong support system of caring friends, family members and health professionals can be highly beneficial. They can bring accountability, perspective and encouragement too. Recovery is a process of exploration; you don't need to do it alone.

Finally, don't forget to celebrate! Each step forward deserves recognition. Write down everything you've achieved so far, no matter how small. It uplifts the path of recovery and honours you as the person who is courageously walking it out.

SPIRITUAL KEYS

Did you know that even in modern society, over half of the Australian adult population aligns with Christianity and another 8.2% with other religions?[33] This makes it likely that a considerable number of people with anorexia have faith in God. Since spirituality can play a central role in informing someone of their identity, worth and purpose, it's vital to grasp spiritual truths so that lies entangled in self-perception can be discerned and undone. So, below, I have counteracted some common faulty beliefs with spiritual truths, which serve as keys, unlocking further hope and freedom.

Anorexia is a sin. Therefore, I am unacceptable to God.

Truth - Regardless of whether or not anorexia is a sin, we all sin, and God loves us anyway (Romans 3:23-24 and 5:8 NIV). Through Jesus' life, death and resurrection, all those who put their faith in him are acceptable to God as they are made new, pure and holy (2 Corinthians 5:17, 1 Corinthians 1:30). Because of Jesus, all our sin (past, present and future) is as far as the east is from the west (Psalm 103:12). So, while it's certainly good to be free from an eating disorder if we have one, it doesn't disqualify us from God's love and eternal life. Nothing can separate us from his love, not even anorexia (Romans 8:31-39).

My thoughts, feelings and behaviours are bad—I deserve to be punished.

Truth - Jesus paid the price for our sins when he died on the cross (Isaiah 53:5). This leaves no reason to punish ourselves. Instead, we can boldly approach God, with all our mess, raw emotions and sin and experience grace, mercy and healing (Hebrews 4:16, 2 Corinthians 12:9). At the same time, our thoughts, feelings and actions may not be "bad." So, it's helpful to talk to a well-trained psychologist or pastor to gain feedback and further truths that set us free.

I need more self-discipline.

Truth - "God has not given us a spirit of fear and timidity, but of power, love and self-discipline" (2 Timothy 1:7 NLT). We do not need more self-discipline because it already lies within. All we need to do is partner with God, who helps us develop and exercise self-discipline and looks after our heart and wellbeing through the process (Galatians 5:22-23, Matthew 11:28-30). Our attempt at self-discipline can be harsh, squash our sense of self and even lead to feeling out of control. Yet walking with God, we can find self-discipline that brings life instead of draining it (John 15:5).

Clean eating makes me pure.

Truth - Wanting to feel clean can point us to a profound spiritual reality and yearning within. Yet it is faulty to believe that certain foods have the power to make us "pure" or "dirty." 1 John 1:7 (NIV) says, "...the blood of Jesus, his Son, purifies us from all sin." Jesus, through the Holy Spirit, makes us clean. No amount of eating "clean, healthy or good" food can do this. Likewise, no amount of eating "unclean, junk or bad" food can undo what Jesus' atonement has achieved. Jesus even says, "Don't you see that nothing that enters a person from the outside can defile them? For it (food) doesn't go into their heart but into their stomach, and then out of the body" (Mark 7:18-19). Moreover, from a health perspective, food is not "good" or "bad," so speaking to a dietitian about this topic can be helpful too.

I am weak if I seek help.

Truth - Seeing a therapist, entering treatment or taking prescribed medication is not a sign of weakness, lack of faith or failure to rely on God. Seeking help is wise. Proverbs 12:15 says, "…the wise listen to advice." Similarly, Proverbs 24:6 says, "Surely you need guidance to wage war, and victory is won through many advisers." What's more, the Bible portrays doctors and medicine in a positive light. The disciple Luke was called the "beloved physician," and traditional treatment was often sought (Colossians 4:14, Proverbs 16:24, 2 Kings 20:7, Luke 10:34, 1 Timothy 5:23 NLT). At the same time, God can and does heal the body and soul, regardless of the interventions used (1 Corinthians 12:9, Luke 6:18-19, Psalm 147:3). He also guides us in all areas of life so we can seek his treatment advice too (Psalm 48:14). The truth is, we can seek help and still look to God for all our needs. Life with him is not black-and-white. It is not medicine or faith. Instead, life is full of colour, freedom and grace.

I am displeasing to God for not looking after my body.

Truth - You are God's child, the apple of his eye. He understands you and your struggles (1 John 3:1, Matthew 18:12-14 NIV). It does say in 1

Corinthians 6:19-20, "Do you not know that your bodies are temples of the Holy Spirit, who is in you, who you have received from God? You are not your own; you were bought at a price. Therefore, honour God with your bodies." However, when read in context, this verse refers to sexual sin, not eating disorders. Regardless of whether sexual sin is also an area of struggle for you, "…there is now no condemnation for those who are in Christ Jesus" (Romans 8:1). The heart of this verse is not to shame but to help people who think it is okay to sexually sin, to change their behaviour, through grasping their immense worth and identity in Jesus (1 Peter 2:9).

I am a failure. I am beyond help.

Truth - Who you are is not based on success or failure, being "good" or "bad," but who God says you are. And he says this: You are chosen and adopted (Ephesians 1:4-5). You are so valuable that the very hairs on your head are numbered (Matthew 10:29-31). You are the light of the world (Matthew 5:14). You are a saint, steward and soldier (Romans 1:7, 1 Peter 4:10, 2 Timothy 2:3). Through Jesus, you are victorious and crowned with love (1 Corinthians 15:57, Psalm 103:4). Who you are in Christ, whether you remain unwell, relapse or recover, does not change. Neither does God's love. No matter how many times you "slip up" or "fall down," God says, "Never will I leave you; never will I forsake you" (Hebrews 13:5). He also says, "Come to me, all you who are weary and burdened, and I will give you rest" (Matthew 11:28). Even when everything may seem hopeless, God is still for you and has great plans and hope for your future (Romans 8:31 and Jeremiah 29:11). You are more valuable—just as you are—than you can ever imagine (John 3:16).

ON REFLECTION

Reflecting on treatment for anorexia brought up many questions for me. Perhaps it has for you too. Should treatment be forced? Should complete weight restoration always be the aim? Should recovery programs be generic or tailor-made? And should treatment help a person spiritually and socially? Even though I haven't found all the answers, pondering these big questions has been beneficial because it has led me to dig deep and question what I truly believe.

Through investigating legal and research articles, I found some, though often varied, answers. For instance, the law allows for situations where treatment can be mandated against someone's wishes.[34] Research also shows that people with anorexia tend to agree in retrospect with the necessity of compulsory treatment to save a life. Yet, they emphasise that treatment must be ethical and caring.[35] Concerning weight restoration, one medical study suggested that complete weight restoration should be the goal for those with both short and long-term anorexia.[36] Still, another research article proposes that personalised treatment is best.[37]

However, I noticed that they often overlooked spirituality as a source of guidance around treatment. Spirituality, for me, involves believing that Jesus is "the God who heals" and empowers people to heal as well. So, I looked closer at Jesus' interactions with the sick and tormented to find more answers to these intricate health questions (Psalm 103:3, Mark 16:17-18).

I found Jesus holistically and completely healed people, and each healing was tailor-made. And although he never forced healing, he did forcefully stand against the darkness that tormented people and relentlessly offered them the fullness of life. The healing Jesus offered also equipped people to re-enter community life, and no one in his eyes was unworthy of help. Everyone was worthy and able to be healed and set free (Matthew 8:1-5, 16). So, by incorporating both my understanding of anorexia and spirituality, I believe:

Personalised, patient-centred treatment that supports complete recovery—body and soul—should be offered, but not forced. Yet, there may be occasions when intervention is needed to save the person from torment and death. At all times, love and respect are to be shown, which includes helping the person spiritually and socially. Through it all, the person with anorexia is to know they are worthy and there is always hope.

No one is beyond help.

NOTES

CHAPTER 3

1. Susan Jeffers, *Feel the Fear and Do It* Anyway (Arrow Books Limited: London, 1987).

2. Jack Canfield and Mark Victor Hansen, *Chicken Soup for the Soul* (Health Communications Inc: Florida, 1993).

3. Sanna Aila Gustafsson, Karin Stenström, Hanna Olofsson, Agneta Petterson and Karin Wilbe Ramsay, "Experiences of eating disorders from the perspectives of patients, family members and health care professionals: a meta-review of qualitative evidence syntheses," 2021, *J Eat Disord 9, 156,* accessed August 9, 2023, https://doi.org/10.1186/s40337-021-00507-4

CHAPTER 4

4. Federica Toppino, Paola Longo, Matteo Martini, Giovanni Abbate-Daga and Enrica Marzola, "Body mass index specifiers in anorexia nervosa: anything below the 'extreme'?" 2022, J *Clin Med,* accessed August 16, 2023, https://www.ncbi.nlm.nih.gov/pmc/articles/PMC8837073/

5. Jenni Schaefer, *Life Without Ed- How One Woman Declared Independence from Her Eating Disorder and How You Can Too,* Tenth Anniversary Edition (McGraw Hill: United States, 2004).

CHAPTER 5

6. Anna Skowrońska, Klaudia Sójta and Dominik Strzelecki, "Refeeding syndrome as treatment complication of anorexia nervosa," 2019, *Psychiatr Pol,* accessed August 16, 2023, https://pubmed.ncbi.nlm.nih.gov/31955189/

CHAPTER 6

7. Richard Foster, *Celebration of Discipline* (Hodder & Stoughton: London, 2008).

8. Rebecca Reynolds, "Orthorexia nervosa when righteous eating becomes an obsession," 2015, *The Conversation,* accessed February 23, 2019, http://theconversation.com/orthorexia-nervosa-when-righteous-eating-becomes-an-obsession-36484

CHAPTER 7

9. Neil T. Anderson, *Victory Over the Darkness* (Regal Books: California, 2000).

10. Nicky Cruz and Jamie Buckingham, *Run Baby Run* (Hodder & Stoughton: London, 2003).

11. John Eldredge and Staci Eldredge, *Captivating* (Thomas Nelson Inc: Nashville, Tennessee, United States, 2005).

CHAPTER 9

12. National Institute of Mental Health, "Eating disorders: about more than food," 2001, *NIH Publication No. 21-MH-4901*, accessed October 1, 2023, https://www.nimh.nih.gov/health/publications/eating-disorders

13. State of Victoria, Department of Health and Human Services, "Victorian eating disorder strategy-PDF," 2014, accessed January 4, 2021, http://www.health.vic.gov.au/publications/victorian-eating-disorders-strategy

14. Tracey Wade, "Epigenetics offers a glimmer of hope for future anorexia treatment," 2013, *The Conversation,* accessed February 16, 2016, http://theconversation.com / epigenetics-offers-a-glimmer-of-hope-for-future-anorexia-treatment-9358

CHAPTER 10

15. Maxine Vorster, *Hidden Hunger- Overcoming Eating Disorders Through God's Healing Power,* Revised Edition. (Authentic Media: Great Britain, 2006).

16. Barbara Mitra, Diana Archer, Joanne Hurst, Deborah Lycett, "The role of religion, spirituality and social media in the journey of eating disorders: a qualitative exploration of participants in the 'TastelifeUK' eating disorder recovery programme," 2003, J *Relig Health,* accessed September 29, 2023, http://www.doi.org/10.1007/s10943-023-01861-0

CHAPTER 11

17. National Institute of Mental Health, "Eating disorders," last reviewed 2023, accessed October 1, 2023, https://www.nimh.nih.gov/health/topics/eating-disorders

18. P. Scott Richards, Michael E. Berrett, Carrie L. Caoili, Sabree A. Crowton, Randy K. Hardman, Russell N. Jackson and Peter W. Sanders, "An exploration of the role of religion and spirituality in the treatment and recovery of patients with eating disorders," 2018, *Faculty Publications. 3840,* accessed October 1, 2023, https://scholarsarchive.byu.edu/cgi/viewcontent.cgi?article=4806&context=facpub

19. Gabriella Heruc, Kim Hurst, Anjanette Casey, Kate Flemming, Jeremy Freeman *et al.* "ANZAED Eating disorder treatment principles and general clinical practice and training standards," 2020, *J Eat Disord 8, 6,* accessed October 2, 2023, https://doi.org/10.1186/s40337-020-00341-0

20. Carrie Caoili, "The role of spirituality in treatment and recovery from eating disorders," 2015, *Theses and Dissertations,* accessed October 2, 2023, https://scholarsarchive.byu.edu/cgi/viewcontent.cgi?article=6483&context=etd

21. Faune Taylor Smith, P. Scott Richards, Lane Fischer and Randy K. Hardman, "Intrinsic religiousness and spiritual well-being as predictors of treatment outcome among women with eating disorders," 2003, *Eating Disorders: Journal of Treatment and Prevention, 11, 15-26,* accessed October 2, 2023, https://pubmed.ncbi.nlm.nih.gov/16864284/

22. Caoili, Carrie, "The role of spirituality in treatment and recovery from eating disorders," 2015, *Theses and Dissertations,* accessed October 2, 2023, *https://scholarsarchive.byu.edu/cgi/viewcontent.cgi?article=6483&context=etd*

23. Rebekah Rankin, Janet Conti, Lucie Ramjan and Phillipa Hay, "A systematic review of people's lived experiences of inpatient treatment for anorexia nervosa: living in a 'bubble'," 2023, *J Eat Disord* 11, 95, accessed October 2, 2023, https://jeatdisord.biomedcentral.com/articles/10.1186/s40337-023-00820-0#citeas

24. Janet E. Conti, "Recovering identity from anorexia nervosa: women's constructions of their experiences of recovery from anorexia nervosa over 10 years," 2018, *Journal of Constructivist Psychology*, 31:1, 72-94, accessed May 15, 2023, http://doi: 10.1080/10720537.2016.125136615

25. Chengyuan Zhang, "What can we learn from the history of male anorexia nervosa?" 2014, J *Eat Disord 2, 138,* accessed February 23, 2020, https://doi.org/10.1186/s40337-014-0036-9

CHAPTER 12

26. Sally Morgan and Ambelin Kwaymullina, *I Love Me* (Fremantle Press: Western Australia, 2018).

27. "Sam Levenson," Last modified 2022, *Wikipedia,* accessed March 18, 2021, https://en.m.wikipedia.org/wiki/Sam_Levenson

AFTERWORD

28. Daniel Akrawi, Roger Bartrop, Ursula Potter and Stephen Touyz, "Religiosity, spirituality in relation to disordered eating and body image concerns: A systematic review," 2015, *J Eat Disord 3, 29,* accessed February 16, 2019, https://doi.org/10.1186/s40337-015-0064-0

SEEKING SUPPORT

29. State of Victoria, Department of Health and Human Services, "Victorian eating disorder strategy-PDF," 2014, accessed January 4, 2021, http://www.health.vic.gov.au/publications/victorian-eating-disorders-strategy

30. Melissa J. Pehlivan, Jane Miskovic-Wheatley, Anvi Le, Danielle Maloney, *et al.* "Models of care for eating disorders: findings from a rapid review," 2022, *J Eat Disord* 10, 166, accessed October 1, 2023, https://doi.org/10.1186/s40337-022-00671-1

31. InsideOut Institute for Eating Disorders, "What are the treatment options?" accessed September 30, 2023, https://insideoutinstitute.org.au/resource-library/what-are-the-treatment-options

32. Margot Rittenhouse, "Effective eating disorder therapy techniques," *Eating Disorder Hope*, accessed October 2, 2023, https://www.eatingdisorderhope.com/treatment-for-eating-disorders/therapies

SPIRITUAL KEYS

33. Australian Bureau of Statistics, "2071.0 Census of population and housing: reflecting Australia- stories from the census, 2016," 2017, *Religion in Australia,* accessed May 17, 2021, https://www.abs.gov.au/ausstats/abs@.nsf/Lookup/by%20Subject/207[1].0~2016~Main%20Features~Religion%20Data%20Summary~70

ON REFLECTION

34. Peter Saul, "Force-feeding anorexia patient curbs freedom of choice," 2012, *The Conversation*, accessed November 29, 2021, https://theconversation.com/force-feeding-anorexic-patient-curbs-freedom-of-choice-7815

35. Jacinta Tan, Anne Stewart, Raymond Fitzpatrick and Tony Hope, "Attitudes of patients with anorexia nervosa to compulsory treatment and coercion," 2010, International *Journal of Law and Psychiatry Elsevier*, accessed November 28, 2021, http://doi.org/10.1016/j.ijlp.2009.10.003

36. Graham W. Redgrave, Colleen C. Schreyer, Janelle W. Coughlin, Laura K. Fischer, Allisyn Pletch and Angela S. Guarda, "Discharge body mass index, not illness chronicity, predicts 6-month weight outcome in patients hospitalized with anorexia nervosa," 2021, *Frontiers in Psychiatry,* accessed November 27, 2021, http://doi.org/10.3389/fpsyt.2021.641861

37. Gabriella A Heruc, Kim Hurst, Anjanette Casey, Kate Fleming, et al. "ANZAED Eating disorder treatment principles and general clinical practice and training standards," 2020, *J Eat Disord 8, 63,* accessed December 1, 2021, https://doi.org/10.1186/s40337-020-00341-0

LET'S CONNECT

I would love to hear from you!

My email is **CassandraAlane@mail.com**

I invite you to check out my website, **www.CassandraAlane.com**

And my social media sites, **www.instagram.com/author.cassandraalane**

www.facebook.com/CassandraAlane.BeautifulLight

www.amazon.com/author/cassandra.alane

Thank you for choosing *Beautiful Light*.